PUBLIC HEALTH IN THE 21ST CENTURY

EPIDEMICS

DETECTING, PREDICTING AND PREVENTING

PUBLIC HEALTH IN THE 21ST CENTURY

Additional books and e-books in this series can be found on Nova's website under the Series tab.

PUBLIC HEALTH IN THE 21ST CENTURY

EPIDEMICS

DETECTING, PREDICTING AND PREVENTING

EDWARD PAIGE
EDITOR

nova
Medicine & Health
New York

Library of Congress Cataloging-in-Publication Data

ISBN: 978-1-53618-976-6

Published by Nova Science Publishers, Inc. † New York

CONTENTS

PREFACE

This compilation first describes several methods for glycoengineering the COVID-19 virus to present multiple a-gal epitopes for the amplification of a-gal vaccine efficacy against SARS-CoV-2 infections. Following this, the authors discuss myopia, the most common ocular disorder worldwide. It is the leading cause of visual impairment in children, and its prevalence is increasing rapidly.

In closing, the authors analyze the importance of the detection and prevention of wheat stripe rust epidemics in Argentina within the context of an integrated management of the disease.

Chapter 1 - The main protective mechanism in humans against viral epidemics is the activity of the immune system which produces neutralizing antibodies that prevent the virus from infecting cells and destroy it. The immune system also produces T lymphocytes that kill cells infected by the virus and thus prevent further replication of the virus. In each infected individual there is a "race" between the replicating virus damaging various tissues and the immune system preventing infecting viruses from reaching a lethal mass. In some epidemics or pandemics, the immune system of many individuals fails to "catch up" with the expanding virus populations, resulting in death of the infected person. The development of vaccines prepared of inactivated virus, attenuated virus, or of isolated viral proteins (subunit vaccines) has enabled the "education" of the immune system to fight effectively the infectious virus by inducing expansion of lymphocyte populations that react rapidly against the antigens of the virus. Thus, upon infection, these expanded virus specific lymphocyte populations are activated to neutralize and destroy the virus thereby stopping its replication and preventing its deleterious effects. However, some vaccines are suboptimal and do not elicit a sufficiently protective immune response in many of the vaccinated individuals (in particular in elderly populations). In a number of viral vaccines the low immunogenicity (i.e., efficacy) is caused by the masking (i.e., camouflaging) of vaccinating viral antigens by multiple carbohydrate chains (glycans) forming "glycan shields" that are not recognized by the immune system as foreign antigens (e.g., HIV and SARS-CoV-2 causing the Covid-19 pandemic). Immunogenicity of such viral vaccines may be markedly amplified by a novel immunotherapeutic approach which harnesses a natural antibody that is produced in large amounts in all humans who are not severely immunosuppressed. This antibody is called the "natural anti-Gal antibody" and the carbohydrate antigen it binds is the "a-gal epitope" with the structure Gala1-3Galb1-4GlcNAc-R. This chapter describes amplification of anti-viral vaccines immunogenicity by modifying the glycans on the glycan shield of the virus, referred to as "glycoengineering." Such amplification of vaccine immunogenicity is achieved by glycoengineering the vaccinating inactivated virus or its subunit vaccine to present a-gal epitopes. Upon vaccination with these vaccines (called "a-gal vaccines), the natural anti-Gal antibody binds to the multiple a-gal epitopes presented on the a-gal vaccine and forms immune complexes with it. The Fc portion of anti-Gal in these immune complexes binds to Fc receptors on antigen presenting cells (APC) and induces extensive uptake of the vaccine by APC, mediated by active endocytosis. In the absence of immune complexes, the uptake is suboptimal due to random pinocytosis. The ensuing extensive transport of these immune complexes to regional lymph nodes by the APC results in 10-200 fold higher antibody and T cell immune response than with vaccines that are not immunocomplexed. This is shown in this chapter with influenza inactivated whole virus and with gp120 envelope glycoprotein of HIV vaccines. Studies in anti-Gal producing mouse experimental model demonstrated a much higher survival of animals immunized with influenza a-gal vaccine and challenged with a lethal dose of the virus, than following immunization with vaccine presenting unmodified glycan shield. This chapter further describes a number of methods for glycoengineering of Covid-19 virus to present multiple a-gal epitopes for amplification of a-gal vaccine efficacy against SARS-CoV-2 infections.

Chapter 2 - Myopia is the most common ocular disorder worldwide. It is the leading cause of visual impairment in children, and the incidence is increasing rapidly. In 2010, an estimated 1.9 billion people (27% of the world's population) had myopia, 70 million of whom (2.8%) had high myopia, commonly defined as refractive error ≥ -6D. These numbers are projected to rise to 52% and 10%, respectively, by 2050. Vision impairment related to myopia has significant effects on a patient's quality of life, including physical, emotional, and social functioning. Pathologic myopia (prevalence 0.9%–3.1%), which confers an increased risk of cataract development, retinal detachment, glaucoma, and even blindness, is particularly devastating. Major economic impact has resulted from the increasing prevalence of myopia. Experts have estimated the loss in world productivity caused by uncorrected myopia in 2004 to have been 268.8 billion international dollars and the cost of addressing this problem to be US $28 billion over 5 years. Myopia is a particular public health concern in many East Asian countries, where the condition affects 80% to 90% of high school graduates. Of these individuals, 10% to 20% have sight threatening pathologic myopia. There appears to be not only environmental but also genetic factors that play a part in development and progression of myopia. Initial research has shown that outdoor activity, sun light exposure, and low dose atropine all seem to help slow down the rate of myopia. It is theorized that visual input to the peripheral retina regulates adjacent scleral growth, and the relative peripheral hyperopic defocus in myopic eyes that remains despite wearing corrective myopic spectacles may be associated with elongation of the globe. Some have proposed using contact lenses that emphasize peripheral myopic defocus—and thus minimize hyperopic defocus—to help decrease progression of myopia. Similarly, there have been promising developments in technologies of lens spectacles to help slow down the rate of myopia. Perhaps the most exciting advancements have been in establishing efficacious dosing and drug delivery of low dose atropine to the pediatric population. The concern for this global epidemic of myopia has spurred intense research efforts, and there are a number of promising avenues for prevention and treatment.

Chapter 3 - Wheat stripe rust (SR), caused by the fungus *Puccinia striiformis* f. sp. *tritici* (*Pst*), is one of the most aggressive crop diseases worldwide that threatens global food security. In Argentina, the disease caused the worst epidemics in 2017 affecting about three million hectares. The occurrence of the epidemics was anomalous, as for 87 years there had not been disease outbreaks of this magnitude. The authors were able to relate the epidemics to the incursion of new exotic strains of *Pst* into the Argentine wheat-growing regions, where the majority of wheat varieties are susceptible to the disease. In addition, the authors estimated the impact and chemical control of the disease in the region. Average wheat yield losses were estimated at 3,700 kg ha^{-1} (53%) in field trials conducted in the epidemic area with a maximum of up to 4,700 kg ha^{-1} (70%) in the seven most susceptible varieties. This scenario represents a challenge for plant breeders, since the vast majority of wheat varieties are susceptible to the new *Pst* races. Fungicides showed to be highly effective in reducing SR intensity and yield losses, thus they have become the only tool for managing SR when planting SR-susceptible wheat varieties. In this work, the authors analyze the importance of detection and prevention of SR epidemics in Argentina under the described scenario and within the context of an integrated management of the disease.

In: Epidemics
Editor: Edward Paige
ISBN: 978-1-53618-976-6

Chapter 1

GLYCOENGINEERING OF VACCINES THAT HARNESSING THE NATURAL ANTI-GAL ANTIBODY INCREASES IMMUNE PROTECTION IN VIRAL EPIDEMICS

*Uri Galili**
Department of Medicine, Rush University School of Medicine,
Chicago, IL, US

ABSTRACT

The main protective mechanism in humans against viral epidemics is the activity of the immune system which produces neutralizing antibodies that prevent the virus from infecting cells and destroy it. The immune system also produces T lymphocytes that kill cells infected by the virus and thus prevent further replication of the virus. In each infected individual there is a "race" between the replicating virus damaging various tissues and the immune system preventing infecting viruses from reaching a lethal mass. In some epidemics or pandemics, the immune system of many individuals fails to "catch up" with the expanding virus populations,

* Corresponding Author's E-mail: uri.galili@rcn.com.

resulting in death of the infected person. The development of vaccines prepared of inactivated virus, attenuated virus, or of isolated viral proteins (subunit vaccines) has enabled the "education" of the immune system to fight effectively the infectious virus by inducing expansion of lymphocyte populations that react rapidly against the antigens of the virus. Thus, upon infection, these expanded virus specific lymphocyte populations are activated to neutralize and destroy the virus thereby stopping its replication and preventing its deleterious effects. However, some vaccines are suboptimal and do not elicit a sufficiently protective immune response in many of the vaccinated individuals (in particular in elderly populations). In a number of viral vaccines the low immunogenicity (i.e., efficacy) is caused by the masking (i.e., camouflaging) of vaccinating viral antigens by multiple carbohydrate chains (glycans) forming "glycan shields" that are not recognized by the immune system as foreign antigens (e.g., HIV and SARS-CoV-2 causing the Covid-19 pandemic). Immunogenicity of such viral vaccines may be markedly amplified by a novel immunotherapeutic approach which harnesses a natural antibody that is produced in large amounts in all humans who are not severely immunosuppressed. This antibody is called the "natural anti-Gal antibody" and the carbohydrate antigen it binds is the "α-gal epitope" with the structure Galα1-3Galβ1-4GlcNAc-R. This chapter describes amplification of anti-viral vaccines immunogenicity by modifying the glycans on the glycan shield of the virus, referred to as "glycoengineering." Such amplification of vaccine immunogenicity is achieved by glycoengineering the vaccinating inactivated virus or its subunit vaccine to present α-gal epitopes. Upon vaccination with these vaccines (called "α-gal vaccines), the natural anti-Gal antibody binds to the multiple α-gal epitopes presented on the α-gal vaccine and forms immune complexes with it. The Fc portion of anti-Gal in these immune complexes binds to Fc receptors on antigen presenting cells (APC) and induces extensive uptake of the vaccine by APC, mediated by active endocytosis. In the absence of immune complexes, the uptake is suboptimal due to random pinocytosis. The ensuing extensive transport of these immune complexes to regional lymph nodes by the APC results in 10-200 fold higher antibody and T cell immune response than with vaccines that are not immunocomplexed. This is shown in this chapter with influenza inactivated whole virus and with gp120 envelope glycoprotein of HIV vaccines. Studies in anti-Gal producing mouse experimental model demonstrated a much higher survival of animals immunized with influenza α-gal vaccine and challenged with a lethal dose of the virus, than following immunization with vaccine presenting unmodified glycan shield. This chapter further describes a number of methods for glycoengineering of Covid-19 virus to present multiple α-gal epitopes for amplification of α-gal vaccine efficacy against SARS-CoV-2 infections.

Keywords: viral vaccines, influenza, HIV, Covid-19, SARS-CoV-2, S protein, glycan shield, anti-Gal, α-gal epitopes, glycoengineering, vaccine efficacy

INTRODUCTION

The key prophylactic protective method against infection by epidemic causing viruses which are transmitted from mammalian reservoirs (zoonotic virus) or from infected humans is immunization with a vaccine that elicits an immune response against the virus. Such a protective immune response is mediated by antibodies that neutralize and destroy the virus thus preventing the virus from penetrating into host cells. This protective immune response also includes T cells that identify and kill virus infected cells, thereby preventing further infection of cells and replication of the virus. Viruses causing epidemics usually display poor immunogenicity, i.e., the ability of the immune system to mount a rapid protective immune response is limited. This is because the immune system fails to recognize fast enough the virus as an invading microbial agent that should be destroyed. In each infected individual there is a "race" between the replicating virus damaging various tissues and the immune system preventing infecting viruses from reaching a lethal mass. In lethal epidemics, the immune system of many individuals fails to "catch up" with the expanding virus population, resulting in death of the infected person. Vaccination of populations in danger of being infected by the harmful virus introduces into the vaccinated individual harmless viral proteins (or genes coding for these proteins), thus "fooling" the immune system to sense a viral attack. This enables the "education" of the immune system to fight effectively the infectious virus by inducing expansion of the lymphocyte populations that react rapidly and specifically against the proteins of the virus (i.e., viral antigens). Thus, upon infection by the lethal virus during an epidemic, the expanded populations of virus specific lymphocytes are rapidly activated to produce antibodies that neutralize (i.e., prevent the virus from attaching to cells and infecting them) and destroy the virus by activation of the complement system to forms "holes" in the envelope of the virus. In addition, virus specific T lymphocytes kill cells infected by the virus, thereby stopping its replication and expansion and preventing further viral deleterious effects.

Some vaccines are not effective enough in eliciting a protective immune response in a significant proportion of the vaccinated individuals (in particular in elderly populations). Among the reasons for this suboptimal efficacy are:

1) *Seasonal epidemics* – Changes in viral antigens in some seasonal epidemics (e.g., influenza) which prevent recognition of the infectious virus by the immune system of individuals immunized with vaccines prepared from a previous season virus.
2) *Low immune response to new antigens in the elderly*- Some vaccines are less effective in the elderly in eliciting long lasting anti-viral protective immune response than in young populations, as demonstrated with influenza vaccines (Webster, 2000; Katz et al., 2004; Chang et al., 2012). Because of these differences, mortality among the elderly infected during the seasonal outbreak of influenza virus is much higher than among young patients. Moreover, the lower immune response to SARS-CoV-2 infection makes the elderly much more susceptible to the detrimental effects of the virus, as indicated by the much higher mortality rate of Covid-19 among elderly than in young individuals (CDC, 2020; Liu et al., 2020). Among the many reasons for the significantly lower immune response in the elderly are the near complete to complete elimination of the thymus (main site for T cell differentiation) in individuals 65 year old or older (Kendal et al. 1980), telomere erosion in lymphocytes, damaged DNA and mitochondrial disfunction (Akwbar & Gilroy 2020). A common clinical example which demonstrates the differences between the potent immune response in young vs. lesser immune response in the elderly is the replacement of impaired heart valves with porcine heart valve in the two age groups. Because of the extensive immune response against the porcine antigens in young recipients, the porcine heart valve

function is impaired in 100% of <35 year old young recipients within <5 years. Therefore, young patients are implanted with mechanical heart valve that requires constant anticoagulation therapy (Wang et al. 2017). In contrast, the very weak immune response against the porcine implant antigens in elderly recipients (>70 year old) enables appropriate function of porcine heart valve implants for 10-20 years.

3) *Glycan shields on viruses* – Enveloped viruses usually have carbohydrate chains (glycans) linked to their envelope proteins. In a large proportion of these viruses, the multiple glycans "camouflage" the virus by forming a "glycan shield" that "hides" immunogenic peptides of envelope glycoproteins (Walls et al. 2016; Yang et al. 2020; Watanabe et al. 2020). This camouflaging results in low immunogenicity of vaccines made of such viruses, or of their envelope glycoproteins, leading to low efficacy of the protective immune response elicited by the vaccine. Suboptimal efficacy of viral vaccines was attributed to the glycan shield masking antigens in vaccines of enveloped viruses such as hepatitis C virus vaccine (Ahlén & Frelin 2016), HIV vaccine (Goulder & Watkins 2004; Lewis et al. 2014) and influenza virus vaccine (Wei et al. 2003; Chang et al. 2012; Wei et al. 2010).

All these shortcomings of some viral vaccines raise the need for developing methods that increase immunogenicity and efficacy of vaccines. This chapter describes a method for achieving this objective by altering (called here glycoengineering) the structure of the glycan shield on enveloped virus vaccines, thereby harnessing the immunologic potential of an abundant antibody in humans, called the natural anti-Gal antibody which constitutes ~1% of circulating immunoglobulins. Experimental studies in mice with vaccines described in this chapter, were found to increase immunogenicity of viral vaccines by 10-200 fold. Thus, it is suggested that the proposed glycoengineering may also markedly increase the efficacy of vaccines protecting humans against viral epidemics.

Viral vaccines are usually of three kinds: 1. Vaccines prepared from the inactivated (killed) virus (called inactivated whole virus vaccine), from its proteins (split or subunit vaccine) or from recombinant viral proteins produced in eukaryote or prokaryote expression systems. 2. Gene based vaccines made of gene(s) of viral proteins that are injected into tissues (usually muscles) of the vaccinated individuals for production of the vaccinating protein by the individual's own cells. 3. Attenuated virus vaccines which consists of virus that does not cause the disease but has proteins that immunize the vaccinated individual against the epidemic causing virus. This chapter discusses methods for increasing the efficacy of vaccines included in the first group above and which are prepared against enveloped viruses. The glycoengineering of the vaccine aims to manipulate the glycans on the envelope glycoproteins to present a carbohydrate antigen called the "α-gal epitope," which is the antigen binding the natural anti-Gal antibody. This epitope is illustrated on the right glycan in Figure 1.

Following the injection of virus vaccines (e.g., influenza virus vaccine) into the arm muscle, nothing happens at the injection site other than internalization of the vaccinating envelope proteins or of the inactivated whole virus by antigen presenting cells (APC), such dendritic cells and macrophages. This uptake of the vaccine is mediated by random internalization of small droplets (pinocytosis) of the suspension of vaccinating proteins or inactivate virus that are in the vicinity of the APC. This uptake is nonspecific and the efficacy of internalizing vaccines into APC is moderate. The vaccinating proteins are transported by APC to regional lymph nodes. The APC further process the vaccinating proteins into small peptides which are presented on MHC molecules. These presented peptides interact with the corresponding T cell receptors (TCR) and activate the peptide specific $CD4^+$ and $CD8^+$ T cells (Banchereau & Steinman, 1998; Zinkernagel et al. 1997). The activated $CD8^+$ T cells proliferate, then leave the lymph nodes, circulate in the body, detect and kill cells containing replicating virus. Activated $CD4^+$ T cells proliferate and function as helper T cells which help B cells to produce antibodies against the infecting virus, as well as secrete cytokines helping proliferation of $CD8^+$ T cells and their maturation into cytotoxic T cells (CTL) that kill host cells infected by the virus.

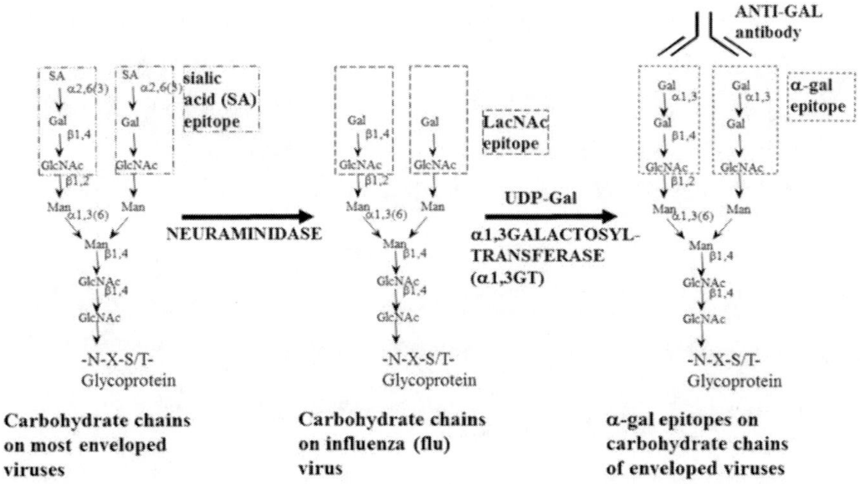

Figure 1. Structure of N-linked glycans on viral envelope glycoproteins and synthesis of α-gal epitopes on these glycans. Left glycan- Carbohydrate chains of the complex type are synthesized on asparagine (N) in the sequon N-X-S/T (asparagine-any amino acid-serine or threonine). Many of these glycans are capped by sialic acid (SA). Center glycan- Sialic acid capping the glycan is removed by neuraminidase to expose the penultimate Galβ1-4GlcNAc-R (N-acetyllactosamine- LacNAc). In glycans of influenza virus the SA is absent because it is eliminated by the viral neuraminidase. Right glycan- Incubation of inactivated virus or soluble envelope glycoproteins carrying the desialylated glycans, with recombinant (r)α1,3GT and with the sugar donor uridine diphosphate galactose (UDP-Gal), in the presence of Mn^{++}, results in synthesis of α-gal epitopes (Galα1-3Galβ1-(3)4GlcNAc-R) on the glycan. These epitopes readily bind the natural anti-Gal antibody, thereby forming immune complexes with viral vaccines presenting α-gal epitopes. From Galili U. *The natural anti-Gal antibody as foe turned friend in medicine*. Academic Press/Elsevier, Publishers, London (2018), page 152.

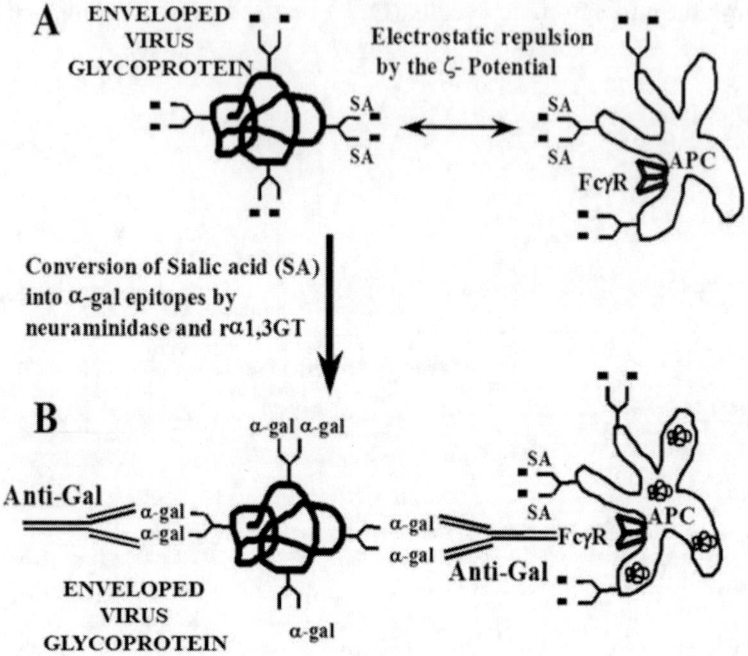

Figure 2. Anti-Gal mediated targeting of vaccinating viral envelope glycoproteins to APC. A. The negative charges of sialic acid (SA) on the glycan shield of viruses and on the APC surface glycans generate electrostatic repulsion (ζ (zeta)-potential) between the inactivated virus or the virus glycoproteins vaccines and the APC. This electrostatic repulsion decreases the uptake of vaccines by random pinocytosis into the APC. B. Glycoengineering of the viral glycan shield by replacing SA with α-gal epitopes, eliminates the electrostatic repulsion and enables binding of the natural anti-Gal IgG antibody to the glycoprotein and formation of immune complexes. The binding of the Fc portion of anti-Gal in the immune complexes to Fcγ receptors (FcγR) on APC induces extensive uptake of the vaccine by endocytosis into APC thus greatly increasing immunogenicity of vaccines. Modified from Galili U. *The natural anti-Gal antibody as foe turned friend in medicine*. Academic Press/Elsevier, Publishers, London (2018), page 160.

One of the critical factors in the process inducing a protective anti-viral immune response by vaccination is the extent of vaccine uptake by the APC. As indicated above, one reason for the suboptimal uptake of vaccines by APC is the random pinocytosis which occurs in many cells and results in internalization of vaccinating virus or proteins that accidentally are near the cell membrane. Another reason for suboptimal uptake by APC is the negative charges on viral vaccines. Enveloped virus vaccines usually present multiple sialic acid residues on their glycan shield (with the exception of influenza virus). Examples for such envelope glycoproteins are the spike (S) protein of the SARS-CoV-2 virus causing the Covid-19 pandemic and gp120 of HIV. The sialic acid has a negative electrostatic charge. When approaching the cell membrane of APC, negative charges on the vaccinating virus or viral glycoproteins and those on the cell surface of APC create electrostatic repulsion (zeta (ζ) potential) that deflects the virus or viral glycoprotein and thus decreases uptake of vaccines (Galili, 2018). Increased uptake of vaccines, which results in increased vaccine immunogenicity, can be achieved by formation of immune complexes between the vaccine and the corresponding IgG antibody. The high affinity interaction between the Fc portion of the immunocomplexed IgG molecule and Fcγ receptors (FcγR) on the cell membrane of dendritic cells and macrophages results in effective targeting of the immunocomplexed vaccine to APC. Binding of the Fc portion of the immunocomplexed antibody to FcγR on the APC generates a signal that stimulates APC to internalize the immunocomplexed vaccine by active endocytosis (Clynes et al. 1998; Schuurhuis et al., 2002; Regnault et al., 1999). The result of this extensive endocytosis is a marked increase in uptake, processing and presentation of vaccines peptides by APC that leads to increased immunogenicity of the vaccine, thus amplifying its efficacy.

Amplification of the immune response following vaccination with immunocomplexed vaccines in comparison to vaccines delivered without an immunocomplexed antibody has been known for ~60 years. Among the vaccines shown to increase the immune response when immunocomplexed with their corresponding antibodies were tetanus toxoid (Stoner and Terres, 1963; Manca et al. 1991; Gosselin et al. 1992; Fanger et al. 1996), hepatitis B envelope antigen (Celis and Chang, 1984), Venezuelan equine encephalitis virus (Houston et al. 1977), simian immunodeficiency virus (SIV) (Villinger et al., 2003) and *Trypanosoma* (Stäger et al. 2003). The immune response against these vaccines immunocomplexed with the corresponding antibody was reported to be 10-1000-fold higher than with the same vaccine in the absence of immunocomplexing antibody. With the understanding of APC role as cells internalizing vaccines, transporting the internalized vaccines to regional lymph nodes, processing them and presenting the immunogenic peptides to T cells with the corresponding TCR, it became evident that the Fc portion of the antibody immunocomplexed to vaccines targets the vaccine for effective binding to Fc receptors of APC, induction of extensive endocytosis into APC and maturation of these cells to professional APC (Clynes et al. 1998; Regnault et al. 1999; Schuurhuis et al. 2002).

The use of vaccines immunocomplexed with their specific antibodies has not resulted in their extensive use in the clinic for several reasons: 1. The antibodies for each of these vaccines have to be purified and complexed *in vitro* with the vaccine. Preparation of standardized immune complexes and the preservation of such immune complexes without inactivation of the antibody are difficult. 2. The immunocomplexing antibodies may be available from non-human species (including monoclonal antibodies) which may elicit an anti-antibody immune response in vaccinated individuals. 3. The immunocomplexed antibodies may mask immunodominant peptide epitopes on the vaccinating antigen within the immune complexes, thereby decreasing the efficacy of the vaccine. The present chapter describes a method for targeting immunocomplexed enveloped virus vaccines and avoiding the difficulties listed above by harnessing the natural anti-Gal antibody. Immune complexes are formed at the vaccination site between the endogenous natural anti-Gal antibody of the vaccinated individual and viral vaccines glycoengineered to present the carbohydrate antigen binding anti-Gal, i.e., the α-gal epitope (right glycan in Figure 1). This chapter describes an experimental model that demonstrates the mechanism and efficacy of this method and the marked increase in the immunogenicity of influenza virus and gp120 of HIV vaccines glycoengineered to present α-gal epitopes. Such vaccines are referred to as "α-gal vaccines." Since this chapter is written ~10 months into the Covid 19 pandemic, the chapter further describes possible preparation of future α-gal Covid 19 vaccines that harness the natural anti-Gal antibody for the formation of immune complexes targeted to APC.

The method for enhancing immunogenicity of vaccines by glycoengineering them to present α-gal epitopes was originally used for conversion of tumors into vaccines that amplify the immunogenicity of autologous tumor antigens (Galili & LaTemple, 1997; LaTemple et al. 1999;

Rossi et al. 2005; Galili et al. 2007; Abdel-Motal et al. 2009a). This chapter demonstrates the use of the same principle in amplifying viral vaccine immunogenicity. Viral α-gal vaccines have not been studied yet in humans. Thus, this chapter includes several figures associated with the studies of α-gal viral vaccines in murine experimental models. The presented results strongly suggest that a similar increased efficacy may be feasible with human viral vaccines glycoengineered to present multiple α-gal epitopes.

The Natural Anti-Gal Antibody Significance in Amplifying α-Gal Vaccine Immunogenicity

The Natural Anti-Gal Antibody and the α-Gal Epitope

The human immune system constantly produces natural antibodies without active vaccination. The antigens (ligands) of many of the natural antibodies in humans are various carbohydrate antigens (Blixt et al. 2004; Bovin, 2013; Stowell et al. 2014). Many of these antibodies are produced in response to antigenic stimulation by carbohydrate antigens on bacteria of the natural gastrointestinal (GI) flora (Wiener, 1951; Springer, 1971; Hooperm & Macpherson, 2010). Fortuitously, a number of these antibodies, although produced against bacterial carbohydrate antigens, also bind to mammalian carbohydrate antigens produced in species other than humans. These antibodies function as an important immune barrier against zoonotic viruses carrying carbohydrate antigens produce in various mammalian hosts (Galili 2020a). One of the major natural anti-carbohydrate antibodies in humans is the natural anti-Gal antibody (also known as anti-α-galactosyl and anti-Galα1-3Gal). Anti-Gal is abundant in human, constituting ~1% of serum IgG, IgM, and IgA immunoglobulins (Galili et al. 1984, Galili, 2013; Hamadeh et al. 1995; McMorrow et al. 1997; Parker et al. 1999). Anti-Gal is also found as IgA and IgG antibodies in a variety of body secretions including milk, colostrum, saliva, and bile (Hamadeh et al. 1995). Anti-Gal is found in the blood of individuals of all ages (Wang, 1995) and is produced as the result of continuous antigenic stimulation by carbohydrate antigens on GI bacteria such as *Serratia*, *Klebsiella* and *E. coli* (Galili et al. 1988a; Mañez et al. 2001; Posekany et al. 2002). When human circulating B cells are stimulated to produce antibodies, as many as 1% of these cells produce anti-Gal (Galili et al. 1993). Anti-Gal is a polyclonal antibody (Galili et al. 1984). In blood-group A and O individuals, anti-Gal also comprises >80% of the anti-blood-group B activity (Galili et al. 1987a).

Anti-Gal binds specifically to a carbohydrate antigen called the α-gal epitope, with the structure Galα1-3Galβ1-(3)4GlcNAc-R on glycans linked to mammalian glycoproteins, glycolipids, and proteoglycans (Galili et al. 1985; 1987b; Towbin et al. 1987; Teneberg et al. 1996) (Figures 1 and 2B). The α-gal epitope is abundantly found on cells and on secreted glycoproteins of all mammals that are not monkeys or apes (non-primate mammals including both marsupials and placentals), in lemurs (prosimians that evolved in Madagascar), and in monkeys of South America (New World monkeys) (Table 1) (Galili et al, 1987b, 1988b). In all these mammals the α-gal epitope is synthesized by a glycosylation enzyme called α1,3galactosyltransferase (α1,3GT), which catalyzes the synthesis of α-gal epitopes by the second enzymatic the reaction illustrated in Figure 1 (Basu & Basu, 1973; Blake & Goldstein, 1981; Blanken & Van den Eijnden, 1985; Galili et al. 1988b). The α-gal epitope is absent in vertebrates which are not mammals, including birds, reptiles, amphibians and fish, implying that this enzyme appeared early in mammalian evolution before marsupials and placentals diverged from a common ancestor (Galili, 1988b). In contrast to New World monkeys, lemurs and non-primate mammals, the Old World monkeys (monkeys of Asia and Africa), apes, and humans completely lack α-gal epitopes because of inactivation of the α1,3galactosyltransferase gene (also called *α1,3GT* gene, or *GGTA1*) in ancestral Old World primates 20-30 million years ago (Galili et al. 1987b, 1988b; Larsen et al. 1990; Galili & Swanson, 1991; Koike et al. 2002; Lanterni et al. 2002). Instead, humans, apes and Old World monkeys, all produce the natural anti-Gal antibody in large amounts (Table 1) (Galili et al. 1984; 1987b; Teranishi et al. 2002). Because of this distribution of anti-Gal and the α-gal epitope, transplantation of porcine xenografts into Old World monkeys or humans results in rapid (hyperacute) anti-Gal mediated rejection of the graft (Galili, 1993; Good et al. 1992; Cooper et al. 1993; Sandrin et al. 1993). As discussed below, a plausible cause for the evolutionary elimination of the α-gal epitope in ancestral Old World primates could be a virus mediated pandemic which eliminated α-gal epitopes synthesizing primates and survival of few progeny in which the *α1,3GT* gene was accidentally inactivated, resulting in production of protective natural anti-Gal antibody.

Table 1. Reciprocal distribution of the natural anti-Gal antibody (Ab) and its ligand the α-gal epitope in mammals

Animal group	α1,3galactosyl-transferase	α-gal epitope (Galα1-3Galβ1-4GlcNAc-R)	Natural anti-Gal Ab
Nonprimate mammals	+	+	-
Prosimians (lemurs)	+	+	-
New World monkeys	+	+	-
Old World monkeys	-	-	+
Apes	-	-	+
Humans	-	-	+

Evolutionary Causes for the Appearance of the Natural Anti-Gal Antibody

Mammals synthesizing α-gal epitopes are immunotolerant to this carbohydrate antigens which is a self-antigen in them and thus, do not produce the natural anti-Gal antibody. Since New World monkeys and nonprimate mammals synthesize the α-gal epitope, it is probable that ancestral Old World primates also synthesized this antigen. The complete lack of α1,3GT activity in Old World monkeys, apes and humans (Table 1) implies that the *α1,3GT* gene was inactivated and thus the α-gal epitope was eliminated in ancestral Old World primates after they were geographically separated from New World monkeys. A plausible scenario for this evolutionary event is the elimination of Old World primates synthesizing the α-gal epitope in the course of an epidemic occurring in the Africa-Eurasia land mass, mediated by a virus that was lethal to primates. However, few primate progeny in which the *α1,3GT* gene (*GGTA1*) was accidentally inactivated by one or few base deletion mutations, survived this putative epidemic. In the absence of α-gal epitopes, these progeny lost the immune tolerance to the α-gal epitope and produced the natural anti-Gal antibody due to antigenic stimulation by GI bacteria. Synthesis of glycans on viral glycoproteins is mediated by the host cell glycosylation machinery. Therefore, virus replicating in the ancestral primates synthesizing α-gal epitopes and killing them also presented this epitope on its envelope glycoproteins. This resulted in neutralization and destruction of such viruses by anti-Gal following infection of progeny lacking α-gal epitopes and producing this antibody. Ultimately, this evolutionary process resulted in complete replacement of α-gal epitope producing Old World primates with primates lacking this epitope and producing the natural anti-Gal antibody (Galili, 2019). New World monkeys evolving in the continent of South America and lemurs evolving in the island of Madagascar were not subjected to this selective process because of the oceanic barriers between them and the primates in Eurasia-Africa. Anti-Gal was also found to bind and kill some protozoa such as *Plasmodium* (Yilmaz et al. 2014), *Trypanosoma* (Portillo et al. 2019) and *Leishmania* (Iniguez et al. 2017). Thus, such pathogens may also be considered as a theoretical cause for the elimination of ancestral Old World primates synthesizing the α-gal epitope and survival of the few progeny producing natural anti-Gal antibody. However, the complete elimination of primates synthesizing α-gal epitopes in all geographic and climate zones of Eurasia-Africa suggests that a virus with very high capacity of spreading throughout populations, is a more likely candidate for a pathogen mediating this selection process this land mass.

Hypothesis on Anti-Gal Mediated Amplification of Viral Vaccine Immunogenicity

The observations above on increased immunogenicity of vaccines administered as immune complexes with their corresponding antibodies suggest that amplification of vaccine immunogenicity may be achieved by formation of immune complexes also with the natural anti-Gal antibody, provided that the vaccines include glycoproteins that carry multiple α-gal epitopes on their glycans. Such an α-gal vaccine in the form of inactivated whole virus may be used as an example. It could be hypothesized that immunization with inactivated virus glycoengineered to present α-gal epitopes will result in the formation of immune complexes between anti-Gal and the α-gal vaccine at the vaccination site. The immunization process by α-gal vaccines is hypothesized to occur in several steps which are illustrated below in Figure 3.

Step 1

Formation of immune complexes between anti-Gal IgM and IgG molecules and the α-gal vaccine will activate the complement system and generate chemotactic complement cleavage peptides such as C5a and C3a which recruit APC, including macrophages and dendritic cells, to the vaccination site.

Step 2

Anti-Gal IgG molecules bound to α-gal epitopes of the vaccinating virus glycoproteins will target the vaccine for extensive uptake by the recruited APC as a result of the interaction between the Fc portion of anti-Gal IgG molecules bound to α-gal epitopes on the vaccinating virus and Fcγ receptors (FcγR) of the recruited APC. This interaction generates a signal that induces active and extensive endocytosis of the immunocomplexed vaccine. In addition, C3b complement molecules formed by the complement activation process and which are attached to the immunocomplexed anti-Gal, further bind to C3b receptors (also called CR1) on APC and generate additional signals that increase endocytosis of the vaccine by APC (not shown).

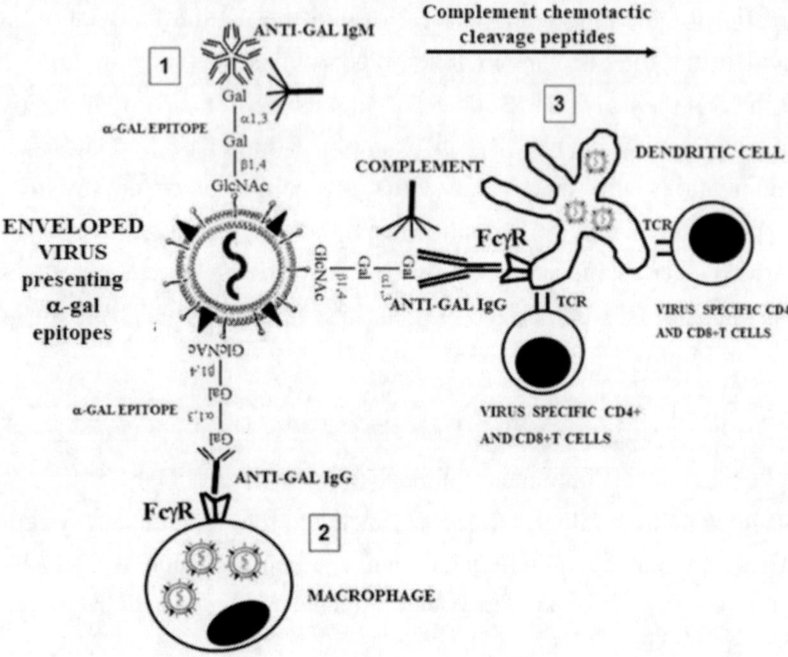

Figure 3. Suggested mechanism for amplification of α-gal vaccine immunogenicity by anti-Gal mediated targeting to APC. Inactivated whole virus vaccine presenting multiple α-gal epitopes is used as a vaccine example. Step 1- The injected virus vaccine forms immune complexes with anti-Gal IgM and IgG molecules thereby activating the complement system to generated complement cleavage peptides C5a and C3a. These chemotactic peptides recruit dendritic cells and macrophages that function as APC. Step 2- Anti-Gal IgG coating the virus targets it for extensive uptake by the recruited APC, mediated by Fc/Fcγ receptors (FcγR) interaction between the immunocomplexed vaccine and the APC. Step 3- APC transport the internalized virus vaccine to the regional lymph nodes and process the virus antigens. Within the lymph nodes, APC present the immunogenic viral peptides on MHC molecules. These peptides engage $CD4^+$ and $CD8^+$ T cells with the corresponding TCR and activate these lymphocytes which proliferate and leave the lymph nodes. TCR- T cell receptor. Modified from "*The natural anti-Gal antibody as foe turned friend in medicine*" by U. Galili, 2018, Elsevier/Academic Press, p. 153.

Step 3

The vaccine internalized within endosomes of the APC is subjected to proteolytic activity of proteases that generate peptides of the viral proteins. These APC further migrate to the regional lymph nodes, process and present the vaccinating peptides in association with MHC molecules for effective activation of $CD4^+$ and $CD8^+$ T cells. The activated $CD8^+$ T cells proliferate, leave the lymph nodes and circulate in order to detect and kill host cells containing the replicating virus. Activated $CD4^+$ T cells proliferate and function as helper T cells that assist B cells in proliferation, isotype switching and maturation into antibody producing plasma cells. Activated $CD4^+$ T cells also function as helper cells to $CD8^+$ T cells maturing into CTL. In the absence of α-gal epitopes on the vaccinating virus, uptake by APC is likely to be suboptimal as it is mediated only by random pinocytosis.

This scenario is applicable to enveloped viruses and to their isolated viral envelope glycoproteins (including split or subunit vaccines or produced as recombinant glycoproteins) which can be glycoengineered to present α-gal epitopes on their glycans. In addition to the enzymatic method described below for *in vitro* synthesizing α-gal epitopes on vaccines, other methods for glycoengineering inactivated whole virus or viral glycoprotein vaccines to present α-gal epitopes are described at the end of this chapter.

Synthesis of α-Gal Epitopes on Viruses

The basic principle in the method of amplifying immunogenicity of viral vaccines presented in this chapter is the glycoengineering of the viral glycan shield for conversion of the multiple sialic acid epitopes into α-gal epitopes in order to prepare viral α-gal vaccines. Many of the glycans on envelope glycoproteins of viruses are asparagine (N)-linked glycans, synthesized on asparagines in amino acid sequences (sequon) asparagine-any amino acid-serine or threonine (N-X-S/T) (Vigerust & Shepherd, 2007). These glycans are synthesized by glycosylation enzymes (glycosyltransferases), mostly in the Golgi apparatus, in a sequential manner resembling an assembly line in a car plant. Part of the glycans are of the high-mannose type having multiple mannose units and the rest are of the complex-type in which many the terminal carbohydrate units are "capped" with sialic acid (SA) as the left glycan in Figure 1. The enzyme neuraminidase (also called sialidase) in the first step (left reaction in Figure 1) cleaves the terminal SA from the SA-

Galβ1-4GlcNAc-R (sialyl-N-acetyllactosamine) carbohydrate sequence and exposes the penultimate N-acetyllactosamine (Galβ1-4GlcNAc-R). The N-acetyllactosamine serves as acceptor for the α1,3GT which links a galactose α1-3 to the N-acetyllactosamine to form the α-gal epitope (second [right] reaction in Figure 1). The galactose is provided by the high energy sugar donor UDP-Gal. The second reaction, which is similar to the one in the Golgi apparatus of cells, is performed *in vitro* by recombinant (r)α1,3GT (Chen et al. 2001). UDP-Gal may be purchased from commercial sources. In the case of inactivated influenza virus vaccine preparation, the envelope glycoprotein hemagglutinin (HA) does not have SA on its glycans. The SA of influenza virus is removed by the viral neuraminidase, thus the glycans of the complex type on HA have the center glycan structure in Figure 1. SA serves as a cellular docking receptor for the HA on influenza virus, and the removal of the autologous SA of the virus by neuraminidase has evolved in order to prevent the binding of HA on one virus to SA on the envelope of another virus. Thus, synthesis of α-gal epitopes on HA of influenza virus does not require the first reaction in Figure 1 (Henion et al. 1997).

Experimental Animal Model for Production of Anti-Gal and Amplification of Viral Vaccine Immunogenicity by This Antibody

The study of the hypothesis illustrated in Figure 3 requires the use of an experimental animal model that does not synthesize α-gal epitopes and thus, can produce the natural anti-Gal antibody. As indicated above, nonprimate mammals including lab animals such as mice, rats, guinea pigs and rabbits synthesize the α-gal epitope and thus are immunotolerant to it and cannot produce the anti-Gal antibody. However, mice suitable for this purpose are the GT-KO mice which lack α-gal epitopes because of the disruption (i.e., knockout [KO]) of the *α1,3GT* gene (Thall et al. 1995; Tearle et al. 1995). Since these mice are usually kept in sterile environment, they lack the GI bacteria which provide the carbohydrate antigens that stimulate the immune system to produce anti-Gal. Induction of these mice to produce anti-Gal is feasible by repeated immunization with xeno-glycoproteins presenting multiple α-gal epitopes, such as pig kidney membrane homogenate (Tanemura et al. 2000), or with rabbit red blood cell membranes (LaTemple et al. 1999). In addition to the use of anti-Gal producing GT-KO mice, GT-KO pigs may be used as a large animal model (size close to that of humans) for studying α-gal vaccines. These pigs lack α-gal epitopes because of disruption of their *α1,3GT* gene (Lai et al. 2002; Phelps et al. 2003) and they naturally produce the anti-Gal antibody with characteristics similar to those of human anti-Gal (Dor et al. 2004; Fang et al. 2012; Galili, 2013b). No other nonprimate mammals have yet been engineered to lack α-gal epitopes. Thus, all other nonprimate mammals cannot produce anti-Gal and are not suitable for studying α-gal vaccines. However, α-gal vaccines may be studied also in Old World monkeys such as baboon, rhesus, and cynomolgus monkeys, all lacking α-gal epitopes and producing the natural anti-Gal antibody (Galili et al. 1987b, 1988b; Teranishi et al. 2002).

OVA Containing α-Gal Liposomes as a Model for Viral α-Gal Vaccine

The study of the hypothesis presented in Figure 3 required the use of a vaccinating antigen that can be detected following endocytosis into APC and which includes an immunogenic peptide of known structure. Such a peptide should be detected by activation of T cells with the corresponding TCR that can engage the presented immunogenic peptide. These requirements could be fulfilled by studying the amplification of immunogenicity of chicken ovalbumin (OVA) as a vaccine model in anti-Gal producing GT-KO mice (Abdel-Motal et al. 2009b). OVA is a suitable antigen for detection of APC internalizing it and for identification of T cells activated by it because the most immunogenic peptide of OVA for $CD8^+$ T cells in mice is the 8-amino acid peptide SIINFEKL (Rötzschke et al. 1991). A $CD8^+$ T hybridoma cell line called B3Z with a TCR specific for SIINFEKL was generated (Shastri

& Gonzalez, 1993). These B3Z cells are activated when they engage APC presenting SIINFEKL. B3Z cell activation can be detected by the subsequent activation of a β-galactosidase transgene *LacZ* under IL2 promoter. Since T cells secrete IL2 as a result of their activation, in activated B3Z cells the IL2 prometer of the *LacZ* transgene activates this gene to produce β-galactosidase. These intracellular activation events occur following binding of SIINFEKL presented on MHC class I of H-2bK^b (called here H-2b) of APC to the TCR on B3Z cells. The β-galactosidase produced following such activation hydrolyzes FITC-di-β-D-galactopyranoside (FDG) introduced into B3Z cells, resulting in labeling the cells by the released fluorescein. This labeling of activated B3Z cells can be detected by flow cytometry.

OVA is a protein that lacks N-linked glycans and thus, it cannot be glycoengineered to carry α-gal epitopes. Simulation of a virus presenting α-gal epitopes, having OVA as a major protein antigen that is targeted to APC by anti-Gal, was achieved by use of OVA encapsulated within liposomes that present multiple α-gal epitopes (Abdel-Motal et al. 2009b). These α-gal liposomes are prepared from phospholipids, cholesterol and glycolipids extracted from rabbit red blood cell membranes. They present ~10^{15} α-gal epitopes/mg liposomes and thus, readily bind the anti-Gal antibody (Wigglesworth et al. 2011). Following the immunocomplexing with anti-Gal these liposomes were effectively internalized by dendritic cells and macrophages. Moreover, 24 hours following such *in vitro* uptake of the α-gal liposomes containing OVA (called OVA-liposomes) by dendritic cells, these APC readily activated B3Z hybridoma T cells (Abdel-Motal et al. 2009b). This indicated that within 24 hours, the internalized OVA in OVA-liposomes was processed and SIINFEKL presented on the APC in association with MHC class I.

The *in vivo* uptake and transport of OVA-liposomes to regional lymph nodes by APC could be studied by subcutaneous injection of OVA-liposomes into GT-KO mice, in the right thigh. A week later the inguinal lymph nodes (the right regional lymph nodes of the injection site) were harvested, minced and the cells within them were co-incubated for 24 hours with B3Z cells. APC processing and presenting SIINFEKL within these lymph nodes were expected to activate the B3Z cells. Such activated B3Z cells could be detected by flow cytometry, following gating for the hybridoma cell size. The activated B3Z cells were detected as cells double stained, green for hydrolyzed FDG and red for anti-CD8 antibody-PerCP labeling all the B3Z cells since they are $CD8^+$ T hybridoma cells (Figure 4A).

Lymph nodes draining the vaccination site in three anti-Gal producing GT-KO mice that were injected with OVA-liposomes displayed high numbers of SIINFEKL presenting APC, as indicated by the activation of 14-24% B3Z cells. In contrast, whereas the opposite (left) inguinal lymph node cells, displayed activation of only 2.5-3.7% B3Z cells (Figure 4A). The presence of multiple APC presenting SIINFEKL in lymph nodes draining the vaccination site area depended on the presence of the anti-Gal antibody in the injected mouse. This was shown with wild-type (WT) mice. As indicated above, WT mice are incapable of producing the anti-Gal antibody, as they synthesize α-gal epitopes and thus they are immunotolerant to this carbohydrate antigen. Cells from lymph nodes draining the vaccination site in WT mice injected with OVA-liposomes activated only 2.2-3.1% B3Z cells. This activation level was only slightly higher than that measured in the opposite leg inguinal lymph nodes (Figure 4B).

The data on B3Z cell activation by APC in lymph nodes draining the vaccination site suggest that anti-Gal mediated targeting of the vaccine to APC greatly increases uptake and transport of the vaccine to regional lymph nodes, as well as the processing and presentation of vaccinating antigens by APC. This, in turn, amplifies the activation of T cells specific for the immunogenic vaccine peptides. The increased activation of T cells could be further demonstrated by ELISPOT with spleen lymphocytes from the immunized mice that were co-incubated with dendritic cells pulsed with SIINFEKL. In this assay, individual activated T cells are detected by their secretion of intereferon-γ (IFNγ) which is captured as a spot on membranes lining cell culture wells and identified by staining with labeled anti-IFNγ antibodies.

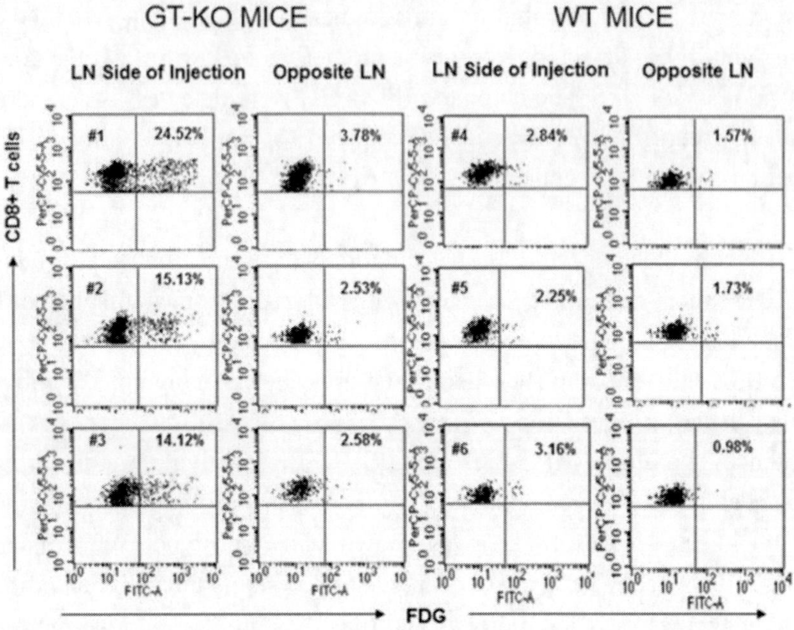

Figure 4. *In vitro* quantification of APC internalizing anti-Gal opsonized OVA liposome vaccine by subsequent evaluation of B3Z hybridoma T cell activation with APC from regional lymph nodes. APC internalizing the OVA liposomes present SIINFEKL on class I MHC molecules and activate B3Z cells. Cells from inguinal lymph nodes (LN) draining the immunization site in the right thigh (side of injection) and in left thigh (opposite LN) were obtained from anti-Gal producing GT-KO mice and from wild type (WT) C57BL/6 mice. Activation by SIINFEKL was detected by flow cytometry of B3Z cells with hydrolyzed FDG. Inguinal lymph node cells were harvested 7 days after vaccination with 10 mg OVA-liposomes in the right thigh. From "*The natural anti-Gal antibody as foe turned friend in medicine*" by U. Galili, 2018, Elsevier/Academic Press, p. 164, after (Abdel-Motal et al. 2009b).

There were on average 20-fold more SIINFEKL specific T cells among splenocytes of GT-KO mice immunized with OVA-liposomes than among splenocytes obtained from WT mice receiving similar immunization (Abdel-Motal et al. 2009b). Accordingly, the proportion of $CD8^{+}$ T cells binding pentamers of H-2b carrying SIINFEKL was higher in the immunized GT-KO mice than in immunized WT mice.

Functional B cell and CTL activities were markedly higher in anti-Gal producing GT-KO mice immunized with the OVA-liposomes than in immunized WT mice that lack this antibody. As shown in Figure 5A, the titer of anti-OVA antibodies (measured by ELISA with OVA as solid-phase antigen) was found to be ~30-fold higher in GT-KO mice immunized with OVA-liposomes than in WT mice after similar immunization. Furthermore, cytolysis of target cells pulsed with SIINFEKL by CTL obtained from GT-KO mice immunized with OVA liposomes was >4 fold higher than cytolysis by CTL from WT mice (Figure 5B). These observations indicate that the elevated uptake of OVA-liposomes opsonized by anti-Gal and the increased transport of the internalized OVA by APC to regional lymph nodes, ultimately result in amplification of both cellular and humoral immune responses against the vaccinating protein. In sections below, the amplification of vaccine immunogenicity is further demonstrated with α-gal vaccines consisting of inactivated whole virus and vaccines containing recombinant enveloped virus glycoprotein.

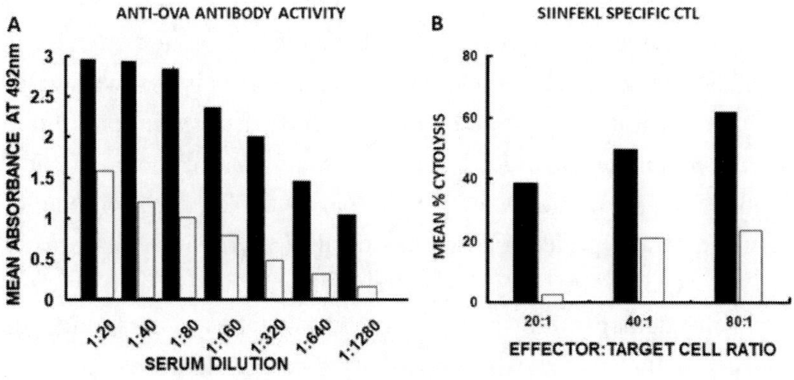

Figure 5. Anti-Gal mediated amplification of antibody (A) and CTL immune response (B) following immunization with OVA-liposomes in anti-Gal producing GT-KO mice (■) and WT mice (□).
A. Production of anti-OVA IgG antibodies was assayed by ELISA, (n=6 per group). B. Anti-SIINFEKL CTL activity with EL4 cells pulsed with SIINFEKL as target cells. Cell cytolysis was assessed by chromium release assay. Results represent the mean of data from six mice per group). Modified from (Abdel-Motal et al. 2009b).

Increased Efficacy of Influenza Virus α-Gal Vaccine

Influenza virus appears around the world in yearly outbreaks that lead to 3-5 million cases of severe infections and >290,000 deaths (Iuliano et al. 2018). The major glycoprotein on the virus envelope is hemagglutinin (HA). The core of the virus contains 8 segments of negative sense RNA, each containing at least one gene. The virus spreads fast by human to human transmission. The HA glycoprotein on this virus mediates adhesion of the virus to sialic acid on cell surface glycans. Based on the annual number of individuals displaying infection by the virus despite vaccination, it seems that presently used influenza vaccines fail to protect as many as 50% of vaccinated individuals from infection by the virus (Couch et al., 1997; Webster, 2000; Katz et al., 2004; Chang et al. 2012). Thus, more effective influenza vaccines are needed to be developed, in particularly for elderly individuals. Development of more effective vaccines is also needed in view of the risk of occasional appearance of influenza virus strains presenting new antigens on the viral envelope HA and neuraminidase. Pandemics caused by new influenza virus strains require the production of highly immunogenic vaccines that will protect individuals of all ages because all humans lack previous exposure to the new viral antigens. This section describes experiments demonstrating as much as 100 fold increase in immunogenicity of influenza inactivated whole virus vaccine glycoengineered to present multiple α-gal epitopes and studied in anti-Gal producing GT-KO mice. The influenza virus A/Puerto Rico/8/34- H1N1 (PR8 virus- adapted to work with mice) was used for these studies.

The HA glycoprotein of influenza virus has 6-8 glycans capped with N-acetyllactosamine (Galβ1-4GlcNAc-R) as the center glycan in Figure 1 (Matsumoto et al. 1983; Kiel et al. 1985). This is the structure of the viral glycans when the virus is propagated in embryonated chicken eggs (lacking α1,3GT). The glycans lack sialic acid because the viral neuraminidase on the virus envelope cleaves the terminal sialic acid off the HA glycans. However, when the PR8 virus was propagated in bovine cells (Madin-Darby bovine kidney (MDBK) cells) or in canine cells (Madin-Darby canine kidney (MDCK) cells), some of its HA glycans were capped with the α-gal epitopes as in the right glycan in Figure 1 (Galili et al. 1996). These epitopes were synthesized on the HA glycans because both cell types have active α1,3GT enzyme (Galili et al. 1988b). Inactivated viruses produced in chicken, bovine and canine cells were studied for anti-Gal mediated uptake by APC according to the hypothesis illustrated in Figure 3. The uptake was assessed by activation of an HA specific T cell clone which has TCR specifically recognizing processed HA peptides presented on the APC. *In vitro* immunocomplexing of human anti-Gal with inactivated PR8 virus presenting α-gal epitopes resulted in increased uptake by APC. This was demonstrated by the ~10-fold increase in subsequent activation of the HA specific T cell clone by processed peptides presented on the APC, in comparison with activation of these HA specific T cells in the absence of anti-Gal (Galili et al., 1996). However, incubation of inactivated influenza virus produced in embryonated chicken eggs, with anti-Gal and APC resulted in subsequent uptake, processing and presentation of viral peptides by APC which was similar to that observed in the absence of anti-Gal. These findings indicated that presence of α-gal epitopes on vaccinating influenza virus enables formation of immune complexes with anti-Gal, resulting in more effective uptake of the vaccine by APC than the random pinocytosis of the vaccine in the absence of α-gal epitopes.

It could be argued that producing influenza virus for vaccine preparation in MDCK or MDBK may suffice for preparation of a vaccine presenting α-gal epitopes that will be effectively targeted by anti-Gal to APC. However, the number of α-gal epitopes on influenza virus replicating in these cells seems to be far from optimal for effective *in vivo* targeting to APC. The number of such epitopes on MDCK cells is ~10 fold lower than that on MDBK cells and may be less than one per glycan (Galili et al. 1996). This low presentation of α-gal epitopes may explain why the efficacy of MDCK produced vaccine is not significantly different from that of vaccine produced in chicken cells (Ambrozaitis et al. 2009; Szymczakiewicz-Multanowska et al. 2009).

Propagation of influenza virus (as well as other enveloped viruses) in available cell lines cannot reach a maximum number of α-gal epitopes (i.e., on each of the 2-4 branches (antennae) of the glycan), because of competition between α1,3GT and other glycosyltransferases (in particular sialyltransferases) in the Golgi apparatus. The last step in the glycosylation process of cellular and viral glycans occurs in the trans-Golgi compartment where in nonprimate mammalian cells α1,3GT and other glycosyltransferases (mostly sialyltransferases) compete for capping the nascent glycan with Galα1-3 to form α-gal epitopes, as in the right glycan of Figure 1, or with sialic acid to form the left glycan in Figure 1 (Smith et al. 1990). The final makeup (profile) of glycans on host cells and on viruses replicating in them depends on the concentration and relative activities of α1,3GT and sialyltransferases (as well as other glycosyltransferases) in the trans-Golgi. Sections at the end of this chapter describes several glycoengineering methods which can maximize the number of α-gal epitopes on vaccinating viruses. One of the methods which has been tried and shown to markedly increase immunogenicity of influenza virus vaccine due to extensive targeting of α-gal vaccines by anti-Gal to APC, uses recombinant α1,3GT (rα1,3GT) for *in vitro* synthesis of α-gal epitopes on the vaccinating virus (Abdel-Motal et al. 2007). The rα1,3GT was cloned from New World monkey cDNA as a truncated gene lacking the cytoplasmic and trans-membrane domains and was produced first in mosquito SF9 cell line expression system (Henion et al. 1994) and later in the yeast *Pichia pastoris* expression system (Chen et al. 2001).

The PR8 virus was precipitated from the allantoic fluid of embryonated chicken eggs by polyethyleneglycol and purified on a continuous sucrose gradient (Galili et al., 1996). The virus was inactivated by incubation for 45 min in 65°C and confirmed for complete inactivation by the loss of hemagglutinating activity with chicken red blood cells (RBC). The virus was subjected to *de novo* synthesis of α-gal epitopes according to the second enzymatic reaction in Figure 1 in which PR8 virus (100 μg/ml) was incubated with rα1,3GT (30 μg/ml) and UDP-Gal (1mM) in the presence of Mn^{++} for 2 hours at 37°C. Control PR8 virus was incubated under similar conditions with inactivated rα1,3GT (10 min incubation in boiling water) and with 1mM UDP-Gal (Henion et al. 1997; Abdel-Motal et al. 2007). The enzymatic reaction resulted in the synthesis of ~3000 α-gal epitopes on the inactivated PR8 virus (referred to as $PR8_{\alpha gal}$), but not on the control PR8 virus. Western blot analysis of the α-galactosylated glycoproteins separated by SDS-PAGE electrophoresis under reducing conditions indicated that the synthesis of α-gal epitopes was mainly on the glycans of the HA_1 molecule, which is the distal portion of the HA molecule (Figure 6). The α-gal epitopes on HA_1 bound both serum anti-Gal produced in GT-KO mice and monoclonal anti-Gal M86 (Abdel-Motal et al. 2007).

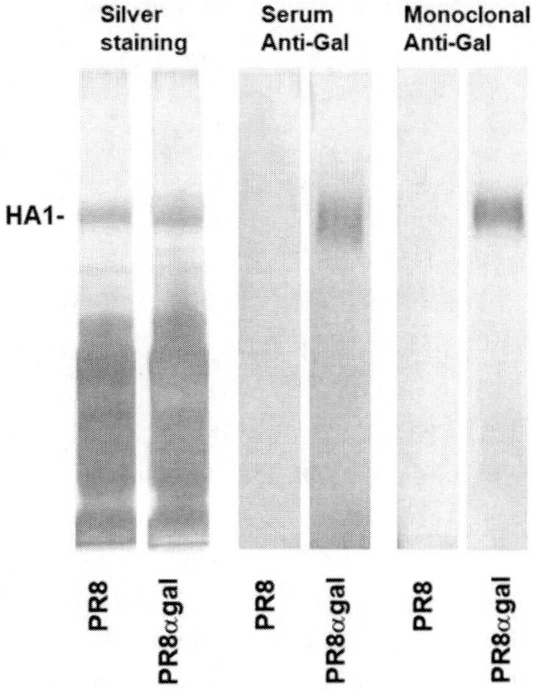

Figure 6. Glycoengineering of PR8 influenza virus to present α-gal epitopes. α-Gal epitopes on $PR8_{\alpha gal}$ were demonstrated by Western blots stained with anti-Gal antibody purified from GT-KO mouse serum and with monoclonal anti-Gal M86 (Galili et al. 1998). Note that both anti-Gal antibodies bind to HA1 from $PR8_{\alpha gal}$ and not to the HA1 from unprocessed PR8. A representative study of three independent studies with similar results. From (Abdel-Motal et al. 2007).

In order to determine whether the immunogenicity of $PR8_{\alpha gal}$ differs from that of PR8, anti-Gal producing GT-KO mice received two immunizations in two-week interval of either 1 μg of inactivated $PR8_{\alpha gal}$, or a similar amount of inactivated PR8 virus. The Ribi adjuvant was administered with the vaccine. The immune response to the vaccine was determined two weeks after the second vaccination. The number of T cells activated by the vaccination was determined by production of interferon-γ (IFNγ) into two types of assays: 1. ELISPOT measuring secretion of IFNγ from individual cells, and 2. Intracellular staining (ICS) measuring by flow cytometry the proportion of cells that are positively stained for production of IFNγ, characteristic to activated $CD4^+$ and $CD8^+$ T cells. In the ELISPOT assay, four of the six mice immunized with $PR8_{\alpha gal}$ inactivated virus displayed ~2200 T cells secreting IFNγ per 10^6 spleen cells, whereas mice immunized with PR8 inactivated virus displayed only ~600 IFNγ secreting T cells per 10^6 cells (Abdel-Motal et al. 2007).

ICS evaluation of IFNγ production demonstrated on average ~21% of cells with positive staining among $CD8^+$ T cells of the four out of six $PR8_{\alpha gal}$ immunized mice vs. ~3.5% of $CD8^+$ cells in PR8 immunized mice (Figure 7A). Similarly, ~13% of the $CD4^+$ T cells from $PR8_{\alpha gal}$ immunized mice stained positively for intracellular IFNγ vs. ~0.1% of $CD4^+$ cells in PR8 immunized mice (Figure 7B). The remaining two mice immunized with $PR8_{\alpha gal}$ (#5 and #6) assayed in both ELISPOT and ICS analyses displayed similar numbers of IFNγ producing T cells as those in PR8 immunized mice (#11 and #12).

The immunization of anti-Gal producing GT-KO mice with $PR8_{\alpha gal}$ inactivated virus also resulted in a much higher production of anti-PR8 antibodies in comparison to mice immunized with inactivated PR8 virus lacking α-gal epitopes (i.e., virus serving as an antigenic source for some of the present day used vaccines). The activity of anti-PR8 antibodies was measured by ELISA in which PR8 virus served as solid-phase antigen attached to ELISA wells by drying aliquots of virus suspension. The titer of anti-PR8 IgG antibodies (defined as serum dilution yielding 1.0 O.D. in ELISA) was ~100-fold higher in $PR8_{\alpha gal}$ immunized GT-KO mice than in the mice immunized with inactivated PR8 virus (Figure 8A). In four of the $PR8_{\alpha gal}$ immunized mice, anti-PR8 production was much higher than in the remaining two mice which also displayed low T cell response in Figure 7.

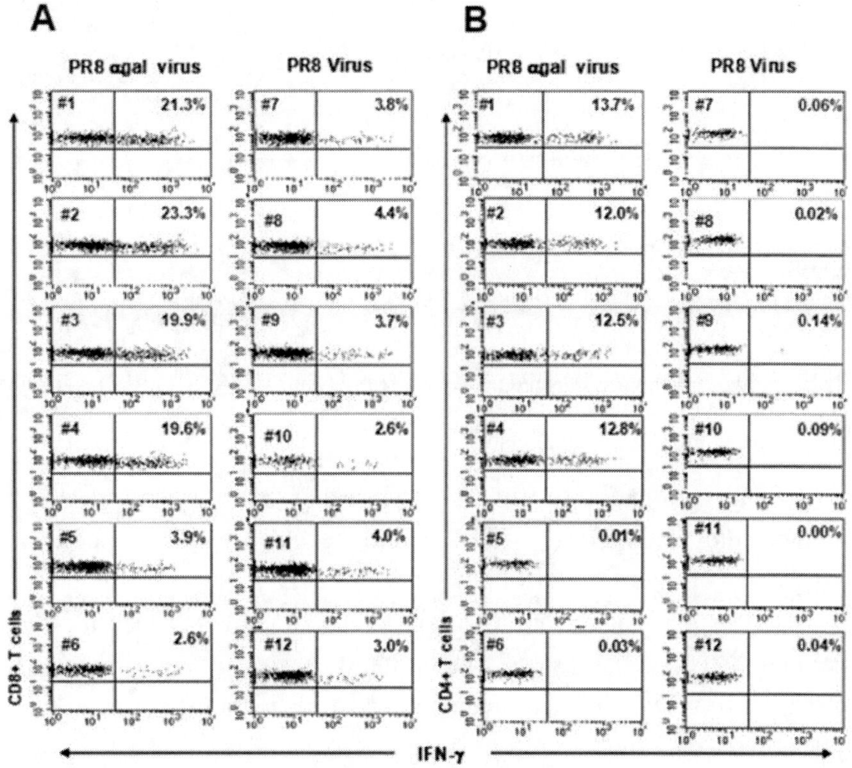

Figure 7. Intracellular staining (ICS) of IFNγ in $CD8^+$ (A) and $CD4^+$ T cells (B) in $PR8_{\alpha gal}$ or PR8 immunized, anti-Gal producing GT-KO mice. ICS analysis in $CD8^+$ T cells (A including two left panels) and $CD4^+$ T cells (B including two right panels) in $PR8_{\alpha gal}$, or PR8 immunized mice (n=6 per group). Lymphocytes were gated in (A) for $CD8^+$ and in (B) for $CD4^+$ membrane markers and analyzed for IFNγ production. Lymphocytes were obtained 14 days after the second immunization and incubated overnight with dendritic cells prepulsed with inactivated PR8. From (Abdel-Motal et al. 2007).

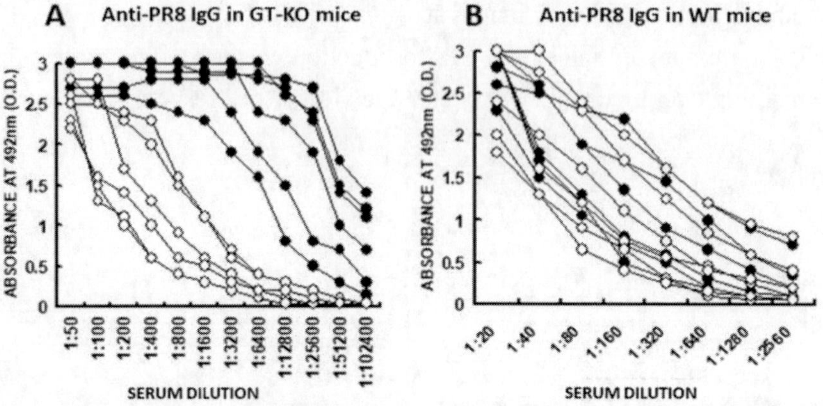

Figure 8. Production of anti-PR8 antibodies in immunized mice. Mice were immunized twice with 1μg inactivated $PR8_{\alpha gal}$ (●), or with 1μg inactivated PR8 (○). Both vaccines also included Ribi adjuvant. Production of anti-PR8 antibodies was measured by ELISA with PR8 virus as solid phase antigen. A. Anti-PR8 IgG antibodies in anti-Gal producing GT-KO mice. B. Anti-PR8 IgG response in wild type (WT) mice. (n=6 per group). From (Abdel-Motal et al. 2007).

The importance of anti-Gal as the antibody targeting the immunocomplexed virus to APC could be evaluated by repeating the experiment of Figure 8A in wild type (WT) C57BL/6 mice. These mice lack anti-Gal despite immunization with pig kidney membranes because the α-gal epitope is a self-antigen in them. No difference in anti-PR8 titer was observed between $PR8_{\alpha gal}$ immunized and PR8 immunized mice. In both groups, anti-PR8 antibodies were produced at a similar low titer that was 80-100 fold lower than that in $PR8_{\alpha gal}$ immunized GT-KO mice (Figure 8B).

The anti-viral activity of these antibodies was further studied by determining the ability of the antibodies to block binding of HA on the virus to its docking receptor, the sialic acid on cell surface glycans. This is performed by studying the inhibition of hemagglutination of chicken RBC by the PR8 virus. The virus was incubated with serum at serial two fold dilutions of the serum. The RBC (1%) were added to the virus incubated in the serum and hemagglutination inhibition was determined after 30 min. Sera of $PR8_{\alpha gal}$ immunized mice that displayed high anti-PR8 IgG antibody activity were found to be >10 fold more potent in inhibiting hemagglutination than sera from PR8 immunized mice (Abdel-Motal et al.

2007). This implies that a significant proportion of the anti-PR8 antibodies produced in PR8$_{\alpha gal}$ immunized mice bind to HA and inhibit its biological activity that enables infection of cells.

The secretory IgA antibody against influenza virus is considered to be the primary antibody involved in protecting mucosal surfaces of the respiratory tract against infection by this virus (Kiyono et al. 2008). Therefore, it was of interest to determine if there is a difference in anti-PR8 IgA antibody production in PR8$_{\alpha gal}$ vs. PR8 immunized mice. ELISA studies for anti-PR8 IgA antibodies in the serum of vaccinated mice were performed by the same method as that presented in Figure 8 for anti-PR8 IgG, using anti-mouse IgA-HRP as a secondary antibody (Figure 9A). These studies demonstrated high titers of anti-PR8 IgA (1:800 to 1:6400) in four of the six mice immunized with PR8$_{\alpha gal}$ that also displayed high T cell response to PR8 antigens in Figure 7 and high anti-PR8 IgG antibodies in Figure 8A. In contrast, mice immunized with PR8 displayed anti-PR8 IgA titers of <1:50.

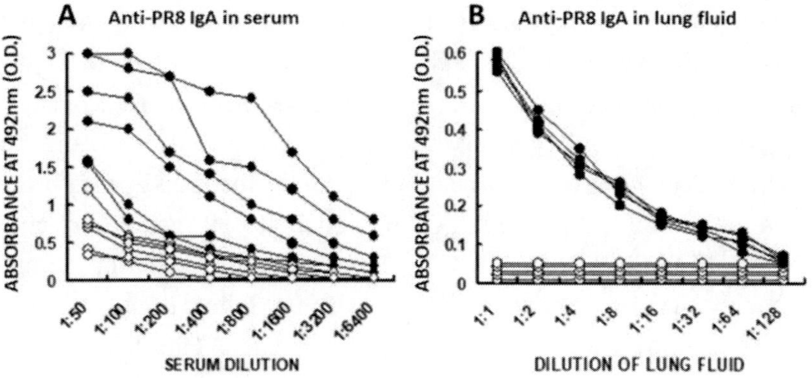

Figure 9. Anti-PR8 IgA antibodies in serum (A) and in lungs (B) of mice immunized with PR8$_{\alpha gal}$ (●) vs. PR8 vaccine (○).
A. Antibody production in the serum of anti-Gal producing GT-KO mice. The two lowest PR8 $_{\alpha gal}$ immunized GT-KO mice producing anti-PR8 IgA are the same as mice #5 and #6 in Figure 7 and also producing the lowest anti-PR8 IgG. B. Anti-PR8 IgA antibodies in lungs of immunized mice (n=6 per group). From (Abdel-Motal et al. 2007).

Study of anti-PR8 IgA antibodies in supernatants prepared from homogenates of lungs obtained from the immunized mice demonstrated the presence of these antibodies in lungs of $PR8_{\alpha gal}$ immunized mice, whereas lungs of mice immunized with PR8 lacked detectable amounts of these IgA antibodies (Figure 9B) (Abdel-Motal et al. 2007). This finding indicated that in addition to amplification of the immune response against the virus within the serum of mice vaccinated with whole virus α-gal vaccine, this vaccination enables the production of anti-virus IgA antibodies that are secreted into the respiratory tract of vaccinated mice. As further shown below, these secreted antibodies are likely to protect the cells lining the respiratory tract from infection by inhaled influenza virus. These observations suggest that the use of viral α-gal vaccines may be of similar significance in prophylactic immunization of individuals against other viruses capable of infecting the respiratory tract such as SARS-CoV-2 that is the pathogen causing Covid 19 respiratory disease (Galili 2020b).

In order to determine whether the antibodies produced following immunization with $PR8_{\alpha gal}$ affect the replication of the virus in the respiratory tract, immunized mice were challenged by intranasal application of 2000 plaque forming units (PFU) of infectious PR8 virus, 14 days after the second immunization. This challenge dose is lethal for 100% of non-immunized infected mice. The mice were euthanized three days post intranasal challenge, lungs harvested and homogenized in PBS in a total volume of 1ml. The virus was quantified in the suspension by measuring the tissue culture infectious dose (TCID) in MDCK cell monolayers at serial dilutions of the supernatant and determining the reciprocal of the highest dilution displaying cytopathic effect. The TCID of lung homogenate in two $PR8_{\alpha gal}$ immunized mice was 100 and the remaining 3 mice had TCID of 10, i.e., lung supernatant dilution of 1:10 was the highest dilution displaying a cytopathic effect on MDCK cells (Figure 10A). In contrast, in PR8 immunized mice, four of the five mice displayed TCID of 1000 and the fifth displayed TCID of 100. The average TCID among $PR8_{\alpha gal}$ immunized mice was ~18 fold lower than that among PR8 immunized mice. Thus, the number of virus particles in the lungs of $PR8_{\alpha gal}$ immunized mice was ~5% of that in PR8 immunized mice, suggesting that the majority of the virus in the challenge was neutralized and destroyed in the former group (Abdel-Motal et al. 2007). A second method of measurement PR8 presence in the lungs was hemagglutination of chicken RBC at various dilutions of the supernatant. The hemagglutination titers (reciprocal of end point dilution displaying hemagglutination) in four $PR8_{\alpha gal}$ immunized mice was 50 and in the fifth it was 100 (Figure 10B). In contrast, in PR8 immunized mice the titer in lungs of three mice was 1000 and in the remaining two mice it was 10,000, thus supporting the TCID observations on the much lower viral load in the lungs of the $PR8_{\alpha gal}$ immunized mice than in the PR8 immunized mice.

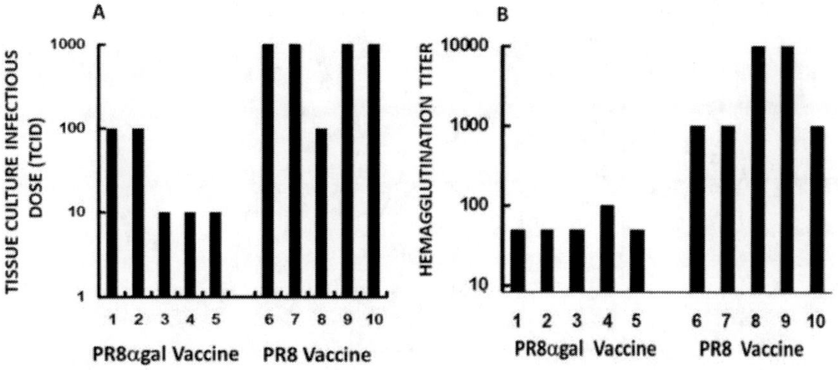

Figure 10. Virus quantification following intranasal challenge by a lethal dose of PR8 influenza virus in anti-Gal producing GT-KO mice immunized with inactivated $PR8_{\alpha gal}$ or PR8 virus. A. Analysis of virus titer as tissue culture infectious dose (TCID) in lungs of the challenged mice, 3 days post challenge (n=5 per group). Supernatants of lung homogenates were incubated in serial 10 fold dilutions in 96 well plates with MDCK cell monolayers. Cytopathic effects were scored after 96 hours. B. PR8 virus titers in lungs of GT-KO mice, 3 days post challenges as assessed by hemagglutination of chicken RBC. The virus titers were assayed in supernatants of lung homogenates (n=5 per group). From (Abdel-Motal et al. 2007).

The ultimate test for evaluating the efficacy of $PR8_{\alpha gal}$ vs. PR8 vaccines is the protection in preventing death of the immunized mice following intranasal challenge by a lethal dose (2000 PFU) of infectious PR8 virus. Survival was monitored for 30 days following that challenge of mice (n=25 per group). Most mice (88%) immunized with inactivated PR8 virus succumbed to the PR8 infection and died by Day 10 post challenge (Figure 11). The survival of three out of 25 mice immunized with PR8 vaccine, vs. the death of all nonimmunized mice infected with the infectious virus implies that this vaccine has suboptimal efficacy, protecting only ~12% of the immunized mice. In contrast to PR8 immunized mice, mice immunized with inactivated PR8$_{\alpha gal}$ virus were much more resistant to the challenge. Only 12% of the mice died following the viral infection and the remaining 88% survived. Survival data on Day 30 were the same as on Day 15 in Figure 11.

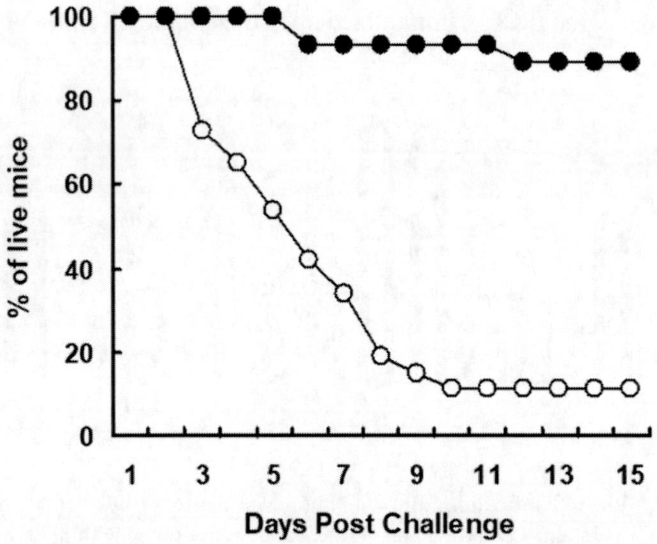

Figure 11. Survival of mice immunized with inactivated PR8 or PR8$_{\alpha gal}$ virus, following intranasal challenge with lethal dose of fresh infectious PR8 influenza virus. Anti-Gal producing GT-KO mice were immunized twice with 1μg inactivated PR8 (○), or with PR8$_{\alpha gal}$ (●) whole virus vaccines. Mice were subsequently challenged with 2000 PFU of infectious PR8 virus, 14 days after the second immunization (n=25 per group). Data presented as % of infected mice at various days. Survival data on Day 30 were the same as on Day 15 post challenge. From (Abdel-Motal et al. 2007).

Overall, the studies with the PR8 virus provide a proof of principle for the hypothesis illustrated in Figure 3, as they demonstrate a much higher protection from a lethal dose virus infection in mice immunized with a glycoengineered whole virus α-gal vaccine than in mice immunized with vaccine of the original virus lacking α-gal epitopes. This higher protection is associated with a higher activation of virus specific T cells and a much higher production anti-viral IgG and IgA antibodies. A recent study has demonstrated increased resistance to challenge by infectious influenza virus in GT-KO mice that were immunized with attenuated influenza virus containing the α1,3GT transgene and thus presenting α-gal epitopes synthesized by α1,3GT coded by this gene (Yan et al. 2020). All these studies suggest that vaccination of humans with virus presenting α-gal epitopes (i.e., α-gal vaccine) may confer a much higher protection upon exposure to infectious virus than virus vaccines that present the original unmodified glycan shield. In view of the current use of several viral envelope glycoprotein vaccines in the form of split, subunit or recombinant proteins, the studies with the inactivated $PR8_{\alpha gal}$ whole virus vaccines raised the question whether a similar anti-Gal mediated amplification of vaccine immunogenicity can be achieved with the isolated envelope glycoprotein or with recombinant viral glycoprotein vaccines. Studies on this issue are described in the section below with recombinant gp120 of HIV as vaccine.

Increased Immunogenicity of HIV-gp120 Presenting α-gal Epitopes as a Recombinant Glycoprotein Vaccine Model

Immunogenicity analysis of an α-gal vaccine consisting of a viral glycoprotein was performed with the major envelope glycoprotein gp120 of human immunodeficiency virus (HIV). This glycoprotein produced as recombinant gp120 of the HIV_{BAL} strain in Chinese Hamster Ovary (CHO) cells that were transformed with the corresponding codon optimized *env* gene. The interest in this glycoprotein stems from the fact that recombinant HIV vaccines trials in primate models and in clinical trials were found to display only suboptimal efficacy in eliciting a sterilizing protective immune response against infection with HIV or with simian immunodeficiency virus (SIV) (Berzofsky et al. 2004; Goulder & Watkins, 2004; Pantaleo & Koup, 2004; Letvin, 2005; Munier et al. 2011). It is expected that an effective prophylactic HIV vaccine should induce a strong protective memory immune response that produces neutralizing antibodies and cytotoxic T-lymphocyte (CTL) response. Combination of these two types of immune response should prevent binding of HIV to its receptors on cells, thereby inhibit infection of cells by neutralizing anti-gp120 antibodies and induce effective detection of infected host cells for their destruction by CTL. Such an immune response should be effective in early stages following transmission of the virus, when the number of infected cells is relatively low, in order to prevent the virus from expanding and reaching a lethal mass. In addition to prevention of extensive virus replication within host cells of the infected individual, a rapid immune response will prevent the virus from undergoing mutations in envelope glycoproteins that enable HIV to evade the neutralizing antibodies without losing receptor binding activity (Wei et al. 2003; Crooks et al. 2015).

Gp120 of HIV mediates binding of the virus to specific receptors. This glycoprotein has 479 amino acids and carries a glycan shield of 24 N-linked glycans of which 13-16 are of the complex type capped with sialic acid (SA) (left chain in Figure 1), and the rest are of the high-mannose type (Geyer et al. 1988; Mizuochi et al. 1988; 1990; Leonard et al. 1990). The glycans of gp120 have a size of approximately ~60 Å, which is ~30% of the diameter of the protein portion of the gp120 molecule in its globular form. Because of the relatively large size of the glycan, the glycan shield comprised of 24 glycans can mask a significant proportion of the immunogenic gp120 peptides, thus resulting in decreased efficacy of gp120 vaccine (Wei et al. 2003). In addition, multiple negative charges surrounding the gp120 vaccine are provided by many SA units capping the N-linked glycan of the complex type. These negative charges induce electrostatic repulsion (ζ-potential) which decreases the uptake of vaccinating glycoprotein molecules, as illustrated in Figure 2A. The protective effects of the multiple glycans of the glycan shield in evasion of HIV from the immune response can be inferred from isolate clones of HIV type 1 (HIV-1) in AIDS patients, where at least half of the mutations in gp120 (i.e., the *env* gene) form new N-glycosylation sites (i.e., Asn-X-Ser/Thr sequon) which increase the size of the glycan shield that protects the virus from neutralizing antibodies(Wei et al. 2003).

All these considerations on the role of the glycan shield in minimizing the immunogenicity of gp120 led to the assumption that glycoengineering this glycoprotein by synthesizing α-gal epitopes on its glycans may increase its immunogenicity according the hypothesis illustrated in Figure 3. It was hypothesized that immunization with $gp120_{\alpha gal}$ will elicit a much stronger anti-gp120 immune response than immunization with the original gp120 lacking α-gal epitopes, as the result of effective anti-Gal mediated targeting of the immunizing glycoprotein to APC.

Synthesis of α-Gal Epitopes on gp120

Glycoengineering gp120 into $gp120_{\alpha gal}$ is achieved by a two-step enzymatic reaction combining the activities of neuraminidase and rα1,3GT, as describe in Figure 1. For performing these studies, recombinant gp120 of the HIV_{BAL} strain was produced in CHO cells and provided as a generous gift from the NIH AIDS Research and Reference Reagent Program. It should be stressed that CHO cells lack active α1,3GT (Smith et al. 1990), although they originate in hamster, which like other nonprimate mammals, has active α1,3GT synthesizing α-gal epitopes (Galili et al. 1988b). It is possible that CHO cells were grown in the 1950s in culture medium containing human serum and the anti-Gal in the human serum selected for growth of CHO cells devoid of α-gal epitopes. Neuraminidase was purified from *Vibrio cholerae* and recombinant α1,3GT was produced in the *Pichia pastoris* expression system (Chen et al. 2001).

The glycans on gp120 differ from those on HA of influenza virus in that gp120 has SA capping the glycan (left carbohydrate chain in Figure 1). In contrast the influenza virus HA lacks SA because SA that caps the glycan in the Golgi apparatus is cleaved off the glycan by viral neuraminidase. The absence of SA (center glycan in Figure 1) enables synthesis of α-gal epitopes by rα1,3GT on the desialylated glycans to generated $gp120_{\alpha gal}$ (second enzymatic reaction in Figure 1). These two enzymatic reactions of SA cleaving and synthesis of α-gal epitopes on gp120 could be performed in one solution containing neuraminidase, rα1,3GT and UDP-Gal, as well as Mn^{++} cations that are required for α1,3GT catalytic activity (Abdel-Motal et al. 2006). Isolation of $gp120_{\alpha gal}$ from the rest of reaction mixture components is feasible by the use of an affinity agarose column with coupled *Bandeiraea (Griffonia) simplicifolia* IB4 (BS lectin). This lectin binds α-gal epitopes (Wood et al., 1979) and thus specifically binds only $gp120_{\alpha gal}$ and no other molecules or ions in the reaction mixture. After washing the column, the bound $gp120_{\alpha gal}$ can be eluted by galactose, α-methyl galactoside, or melibiose solution passed through the column. The specific binding of both human anti-Gal and mouse anti-Gal to the $gp120_{\alpha gal}$ and not to the original gp120 is shown in Figure 16 in the section discussing the similarities between human and mouse anti-Gal antibodies regarding their ability to bind to α-gal viral vaccines.

Amplification of Anti-HIV Immune Response Following Immunization with $gp120_{\alpha gal}$ vs. gp120 Vaccines

As in the studies above on $PR8_{\alpha gal}$ and α-gal OVA-liposomes, the analysis of $gp120_{\alpha gal}$ immunogenicity vs. that of gp120 was performed in anti-Gal producing GT-KO mice. These mice were immunized subcutaneously twice with 5μg gp120 or $gp120_{\alpha gal}$ and Ribi adjuvant, in 2 week interval (Abdel-Motal et al. 2006). The immune response was evaluated 17 days after the second immunization. Assessment of the gp120 specific T cell response in the immunized mice was determined by quantification of IFNγ secreting activated T cells among splenocytes co-incubated with dendritic cells pulsed with gp120 in a 24 hour ELISPOT assay. Each T cell secreting IFNγ is detected as a spot in this assay since the secreted IFNγ binds to anti-IFNγ coating membranes lining the wells and is subsequently identified by a labeled anti-IFNγ-peroxidase antibody. The clear visual difference in the number of spots generated by this T cell activation is demonstrated in Figure 12A which shows the triplicate wells with splenocytes from three representative mice per each group.

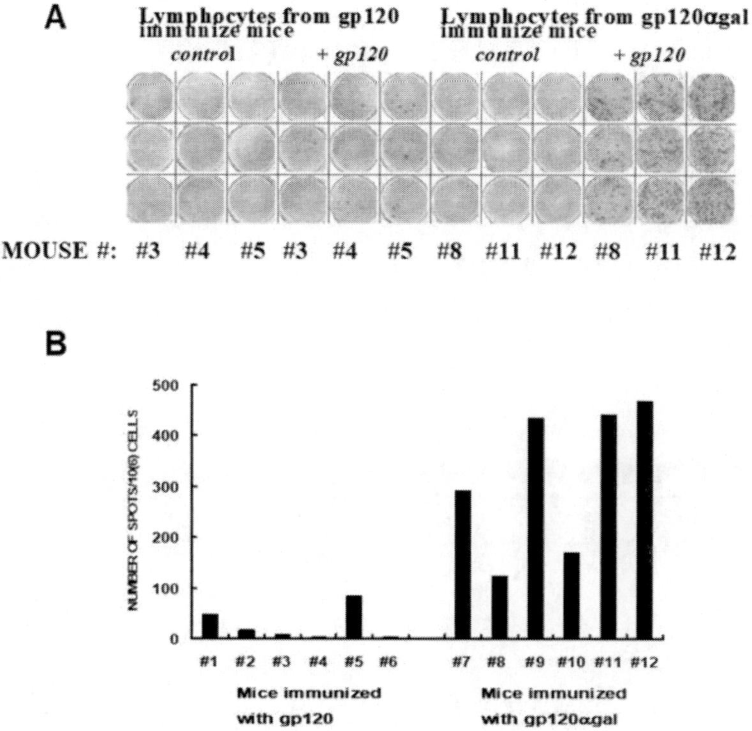

Figure 12. Identification of gp120 specific T cells in anti-Gal producing GT-KO mice immunized with gp120, or $gp120_{\alpha gal}$ as assessed by ELISPOT analysis for IFNγ secretion. A. Photos of spots in wells with splenocytes from three mice, each tested in triplicates wells (vertical lanes) which lacked (control wells) or contained gp120 pulsed dendritic cells. B. Mean number of spots per well from six individual mice in each of the two groups (mean of spots in triplicate wells for each mouse). Modified from (Abdel-Motal et al. 2006).

Practically, no spots indicating spontaneous secretion of IFNγ were observed in the absence of pulsing gp120 as the *in vitro* stimulatory antigen. However, in the presence of gp120 as the activating antigen in the ELISPOT wells, the numbers of IFNγ secreting T cells in $gp120_{\alpha gal}$ immunized mice were visually much higher than those in gp120 immunized mice (Figure 12A). Figure 12B describes the average number of spots representing activated T cells secreting IFNγ in the 6 mice evaluated in each group. Whereas mice immunized with gp120 displayed on average 23 spots (i.e., 23 gp120 specific activated T cells per 10^6 cells incubated in each well in the presence of gp120), mice immunized with gp120$_{\alpha gal}$ displayed ~15 fold higher number of gp120 specific activated T cells, i.e., 332 spots per 10^6 cells (Abdel-Motal et al. 2006).

In addition to the higher gp120 specific T cell activation following immunization with gp120$_{\alpha gal}$, the antibody production against gp120 was much higher post immunization with gp120$_{\alpha gal}$ than post immunization with the original gp120 lacking α-gal epitopes. Production of anti-gp120 antibody was measured in 5 mice in each group by ELISA with gp120 as solid-phase antigen. The vast difference in production of anti-gp120 IgG antibodies is clearly observed in Figure 13A.

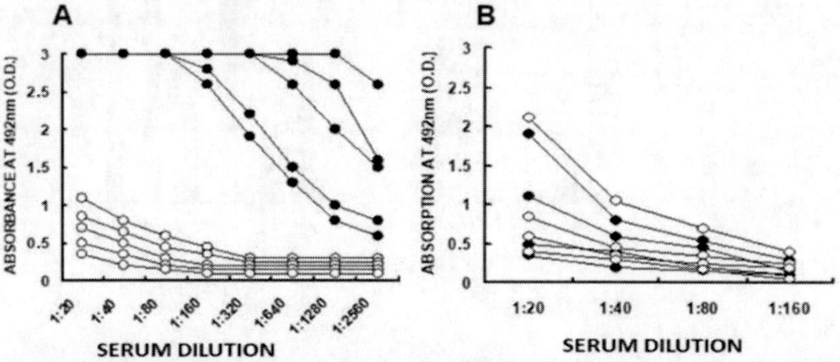

Figure 13. Anti-gp120 IgG production in mice following immunization with gp120 (○) or gp120$_{\alpha gal}$ (●). A. Anti-gp120 antibody production in anti-Gal producing GT-KO mice immunized twice with either 5μg gp120 vaccine, or with 5μg gp120$_{\alpha gal}$ vaccine. B. Anti-gp120 antibody production in wild type mice (WT) immunized as in Figure 13A. From (Abdel-Motal et al. 2006).

Anti-gp120 antibody activity in mice immunized with gp120$_{\alpha gal}$ was 100-200 fold higher than in mice immunized with gp120 (Abdel-Motal et al. 2006). The much higher production of anti-gp120 antibodies was dependent on the presence of the anti-Gal antibody which forms immune complexes with gp120$_{\alpha gal}$ and not with gp120. This is demonstrated in Figure 13B in which the same vaccination as in Figure 13A was performed in wild-type (WT) mice which lack the anti-Gal antibody despite repeated immunizations with pig kidney membranes. All groups received a similar number of immunizations with pig kidney membranes homogenate for eliciting anti-

Gal production. Anti-gp120 antibody production in WT mice was low and similar in both groups of mice indicating that the presence of α-gal epitopes on the immunizing $gp120_{\alpha gal}$ vaccine resulted in no amplification of the antibody response in the absence of anti-Gal. A similar marked increase in antibody and T cell response was observed with antibodies to bovine serum albumin (BSA) in GT-KO mice immunized with $BSA_{\alpha gal}$ in comparison to those immunized with BSA, as well as with CTL killing tumor cells presenting viral antigens (Benatuil et al. 2005).

The ultimate objective of vaccination for production of anti-gp120 antibodies is protection of the vaccinated individuals by antibodies that can neutralize HIV, thus preventing HIV infection of host cells. The neutralizing potential of anti-gp120 antibodies produced in mice immunized with $gp120_{\alpha gal}$ was determined in comparison to antibodies produced in gp120 immunized mice. For this study, the HIV-1 lab strain MN was tested for infectivity of cells following incubation with sera from the two groups, at serial dilutions of the sera. The extent of neutralization was measured by the prevention of T cell killing by the HIV_{MN} in a killing assay of the human T-cell lymphoma line MT-2 infected by the virus (Montefiori et al. 1996; Wang et al. 2005). The HIV_{MN} virus used for mediating killing of the infected T cells is a strain which is convenient for work in the lab and its gp120 amino acid sequence differs by only few amino acids from that of gp120 of HIV_{BAL} (the source for the vaccinating gp120). Thus, it is assumed that anti-gp120 antibodies mediated prevention of MT-2 cell killing by HIV_{MN} would serve as a positive conservative result on even higher neutralizing effect of the anti-gp120 antibodies on HIV_{BAL} infecting T cells.

In accord with the low titers of anti-gp120 antibodies in sera of mice immunized with gp120 (Figure 13A), these sera displayed no neutralizing activity above that of the nonimmunized mice (mice #1 to #6 in Figure 14). In contrast, antibodies in sera of mice immunized with $gp120_{\alpha gal}$ (mice #7 to #12 in Figure 14) were found to display very effective neutralization activities, which were similar to that observed in the positive control of rabbit serum containing anti-HIV neutralizing antibodies (originating from a rabbit receiving multiple immunizations with gp120) (Wang et al., 2005).

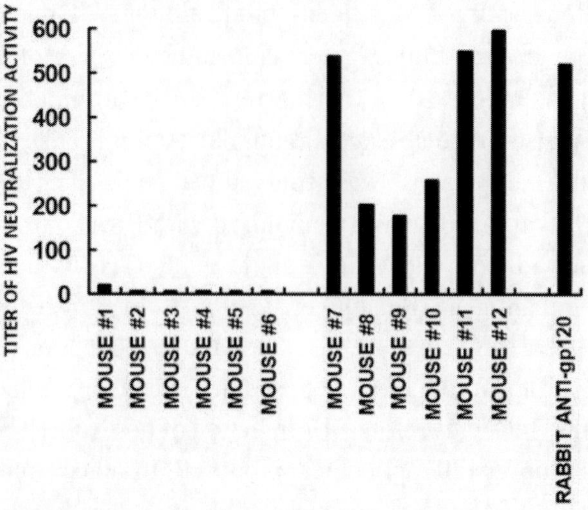

Figure 14. Evaluation of neutralizing antibody activity in anti-Gal producing GT-KO mice. Mice were immunized with gp120 (mice #1-#6), or with gp120$_{\alpha gal}$ (mice #7-#12). Titer is defined as reciprocal of serum dilution displaying 50% neutralization. From (Abdel-Motal et al. 2006).

These results demonstrate a correlation between the high titer of anti-gp120 antibody production as a result of immunization with gp120$_{\alpha gal}$ and the neutralizing activity of the elicited antibodies. Overall, the findings on the immune response in mice immunized with gp120$_{\alpha gal}$ vs. mice immunized with gp120 suggest that both T cell activation against the gp120 peptides and antibody production against gp120 are much higher in mice that were immunized with recombinant envelope glycoprotein α-gal vaccine than in mice immunized with recombinant envelope glycoprotein vaccine lacking α-gal epitopes. These findings are in line with the vaccine studies using a whole inactivated influenza virus vaccine glycoengineered to present α-gal epitopes. These results raise the possibility that glycoengineering of inactivated whole virus, subunit glycoprotein, and of recombinant viral glycoprotein vaccines for their conversion into α-gal vaccines may serve as a general method for increasing viral vaccine immunogenicity by altering their glycan shield from part of the envelope glycoprotein that protects the virus against the immune system to a component of the vaccine that effectively targets it to APC by immunocomplexing with the natural anti-Gal antibody.

Targeting of Low Immunogenicity HIV Proteins to APC by Fusion with gp120$_{\alpha Gal}$

Studies on possible changes in HIV in the course of infection in humans demonstrated the occurrence of mutations in the envelope glycoprotein gp120 which enable the virus to evade the neutralizing and destructive effects of antibodies produced against the virus replicating in the patients (Wei et al. 2003; Crooks et al. 2015). Therefore, it is assumed that vaccination only with gp120 may not elicit an immune response against HIV infections that is effective enough to protect large populations against human to human transmission of this virus (Goulder and Watkins, 2004; Lewis et al. 2014). In contrast, the internal proteins of HIV, such as tat, rev, p17 or p24, do not mutate in course of HIV infection, probably because of functional constraints that prevent viruses with such mutations from further replication. Thus, these internal proteins may serve as effective vaccines that elicit a cellular immune response which can destroy HIV infected cells by CTL. It has been assumed that increased immunogenicity of vaccinating internal HIV proteins may be achieved by effective targeting of such vaccines to APC. These proteins cannot be glycoengineered to present α-gal epitopes because they carry no glycans. Thus, it was hypothesized that fusion of such internal proteins with gp120 and subsequent glycoengineering of the gp120 glycans to present α-gal epitopes may result in increased targeting to APC of internal protein fused to glycoengineered gp120 (Abdel-Motal et al. 2010). In order to test this assumption, the core (capsid) protein p24 was chosen as a model protein and was fused with gp120. The fused gp120/p24 protein was produced as a recombinant protein in a mammalian cell expression system and the glycan shield of the gp120 portion of the fused protein was engineered into presenting α-gal epitopes by the use of neuraminidase and rα1,3GT, as described above and in Figure 1, thus generating $gp120_{\alpha gal}/p24$ vaccine.

Production and Immunogenicity of $gp120_{\alpha gal}/p24$ Vaccine

In order to produce a fusion protein between gp120 and p24, the gene regions of *env* coding for gp120 and of *gag* coding for p24 were ligated as shown in Figure 15A (Abdel-Motal et al., 2010). The fused gene was inserted into a plasmid downstream from the strong CMV promoter. The fused gp120/p24 gene within the plasmid underwent transient transfection in human 293 cells which produced the gp120/p24 fusion protein in a secreted form. Following the isolation of the fusion protein from the culture medium by precipitation with ammonium sulfate, gp120/p24 was subjected to the two step enzymatic reaction with neuraminidase and rα1,3GT as illustrated in Figure 1. This synthesizes α-gal epitopes on the glycan shield of the fusion protein, thereby converting it into $gp120_{\alpha gal}/p24$. As indicated above, the p24 portion of the fusion protein lacks N-linked glycans and thus it lacks α-gal epitopes.

The immunogenicity of $gp120_{\alpha gal}/p24$ was compared to that of gp120/p24 by immunizing two groups of anti-Gal producing GT-KO mice with each of these two vaccines. Mice received two subcutaneous immunizations of gp120/p24 or $gp120_{\alpha gal}/p24$ in two-week interval. The vaccines were delivered at 5μg per injection with Ribi adjuvant. Two weeks after the second immunization the spleens of the mice were harvested and the splenocytes isolated from these spleens. The presence of T cells specific to p24 was determined by incubation with the p24 immunodominant peptide $p24_{189\text{-}207}$ (Qiu et al. 1999) which pulsed APC among the splenocytes. T cells with TCR specific to this peptide were activated within 24 hour coincubation with the APC pulsed with $p24_{189\text{-}207}$ and secreted IFNγ that could be detected for individual activated T cells by the ELISPOT assay. The number of T cells secreting IFNγ among lymphocytes from $gp120_{\alpha gal}/p24$ immunized mice was ~12 fold higher than the number of these cells in gp120/p24 immunized mice (Abdel-Motal et al., 2010). The proportion of p24 specific $CD8^+$ T cells (T cells becoming CTL) was determined by double staining of cells binding anti-CD8 antibody and displaying intracellular staining of IFNγ. As shown in Figure 15B, mice immunized with $gp120_{\alpha gal}$/p24 displayed 5-20-fold higher number of $CD8^+$ T cells with detectable production of IFNγ than mice immunized with gp120/p24 lacking α-gal epitopes. These findings imply that anti-Gal immunocomplexed with $gp120_{\alpha gal}$/p24 indeed markedly increased the immunogenicity of p24 in comparison to immunogenicity of p24 in the gp120/p24 fusion protein, probably because of the effective targeting to APC of the fused protein via Fc/Fc receptor interaction.

Studies above demonstrated increased immunogenicity of $gp120_{\alpha gal}$ in comparison to gp120 (Figure 13A). Accordingly, immunization of anti-Gal producing mice with $gp120_{\alpha gal}$/p24 vaccine also resulted in marked increase in the antibody response against the gp120 portion of this fusion molecule in comparison to anti-gp120 antibody production in mice immunized with gp120/p24 vaccine. This could be demonstrated by ELISA with gp120 as solid-phase antigen in which anti-gp120 antibody titer in mice immunized with $gp120_{\alpha gal}$/p24 was ~30-fold higher than that measured in mice immunized with gp120/p24 vaccine (Figure 15C). These observations strongly suggest that the use of a fusion protein as α-gal vaccine in which only gp120 portion has α-gal epitopes, results in anti-Gal mediated increase in immunogenicity of both gp120 and p24, despite the lack of glycans on p24. The studies with the gp120/p24 fusion protein further suggest that in addition to increasing the immunogenicity of gp120 by converting it into $gp120_{\alpha gal}$, this envelope glycoprotein of HIV may also serve as an effective platform for targeting to APC other internal virus matrix or core proteins thereby amplifying their immunogenicity.

Based on the presence of 13-16 complex type glycans on gp120 and the 2-4 antennae on each glycan, it is estimated that glycoengineering of gp120 by the enzymatic reactions described in Figure 1 could results in synthesis of 30-40 α-gal epitopes per molecule.

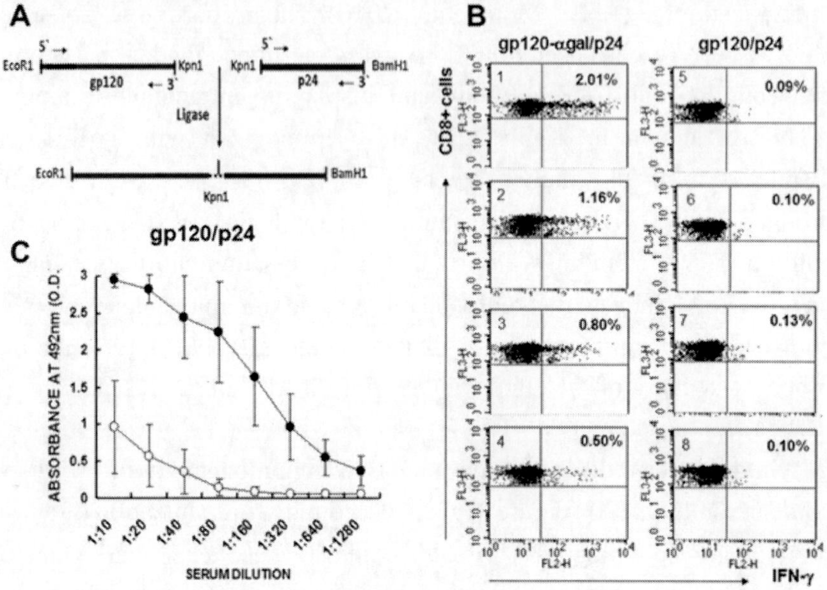

Figure 15. Studies on gp120/p24 fusion protein as vaccine in anti-Gal producing GT-KO mice. A. Illustration of fusion of the genes used for production of gp120/p24. B. Analysis of intracellular staining (ICS) by flow cytometry of IFNγ production in $CD8^+$ T cells specific for p24 among splenocytes of mice immunized with $gp120_{\alpha gal}$/p24 (left panels, mice #1 - #4) and mice immunized with gp120/p24 (right panels, mice #5 - #8). The splenocytes were co-incubated for 6 hours with APC pulsed with p24 peptides. C. Production of anti-gp120 IgG antibodies in GT-KO mice immunized with $gp120_{\alpha gal}$/p24 (●), or with gp120/p24 (○), as measured by ELISA with gp120 solid-phase antigen. Mean ± SD of results from 5 mice per group. From "*The natural anti-Gal antibody as foe turned friend in medicine*" by U. Galili, 2018, Elsevier/Academic Press, p. 164, after (Abdel-Motal et al. 2010).

This number of α-gal epitopes is likely to ensure effective immunocomplexing of anti-Gal with the fusion protein and targeting of the fusion α-gal vaccine to APC. This method for generating fusion proteins between an envelope glycoprotein and a non-glycosylated viral internal protein may serve as a general method for preparation of recombinant vaccinating fusion glycoproteins that elicit effective protective antibody response against envelope glycoproteins and T cell response against both envelope glycoproteins and non-mutating proteins in other viral infections. One example which may be considered is production of influenza virus vaccines containing a fusion protein between HA and the M2 proton channel, since M2 is nearly invariant in all influenza A strains (Fiers et al. 2004; Estrada LD & Schultz-Cherry, 2019). A fusion vaccine of $HA_{\alpha gal}$/M2 may be protective even against infections with influenza virus in which the HA is mutated, because of the anti-M2 effective immune response due to effective targeting of M2 to APC by the $HA_{\alpha gal}$ portion of such α-gal fusion vaccine. Another plausible example is Covid 19 fusion α-gal vaccines comprised of the S protein envelope glycoprotein of SARS-CoV-2 fused with other envelope or internal proteins and glycoengineering the fusion protein to present multiple α-gal epitopes. Suggested methods for preparation of α-gal SARS-CoV-2 vaccines are discussed in sections below.

SIMILARITIES BETWEEN MOUSE AND HUMAN ANTI-GAL ANTIBODIES

In order to determine whether the studies in GT-KO mice described in this chapter are applicable to humans, it is important to examine the question of similarities between the anti-Gal antibody naturally produced in humans and the anti-Gal antibody elicited in GT-KO mice as a result for several immunizations with wild type pig kidney membrane homogenate. The similarities between human and mouse anti-Gal are as follows:

- *Similarity in anti-Gal titers* – Anti-Gal IgG activity was measured in parallel in human sera and in sera of GT-KO mice immunized with pig kidney membrane homogenate. The analysis was performed by ELISA in which synthetic α-gal epitopes linked to bovine serum albumin (BSA) served as solid phase antigen. Sera from both sources displayed similar anti-Gal binding to α-gal-BSA with half maximum binding at serum dilutions of 1:160-1:320 (Figure 16A) (Abdel-Motal et al. 2006).

- *Binding to glycoengineered vaccine* – Human and mouse anti-Gal were studied for binding to gp120$_{\alpha gal}$ of HIV in order to determine whether both antibodies bind to α-gal epitopes. As shown in Figure 16B, both original recombinant gp120 and gp120$_{\alpha gal}$ display the same size since the replacement of SA on the original gp120 with galactose linked α1-3 to the glycan in gp120$_{\alpha gal}$ does not significantly alter the size of this HIV glycoprotein. Both human and mouse anti-Gal bind to the α-gal epitopes on gp120$_{\alpha gal}$ but do not bind to glycans on gp120 as demonstrated in Western blot staining with these antibodies (Figure 16B). The presence of α-gal epitopes on gp120$_{\alpha gal}$ but not on gp120 is further validated by binding of the lectin *Bandeiraea simplicifolia* IB4 to the α-gal epitopes on gp120$_{\alpha gal}$ (Abdel-Motal et al. 2006; Wood et al. 1979).
- *Destruction of enveloped viruses by human anti-Gal antibody* – The demonstration of human anti-Gal binding to viral glycoproteins presenting α-gal epitopes is further supported by several studies demonstrating binding of anti-Gal in human serum to a variety of viruses presenting α-gal epitopes and induction of complement dependent virolysis as a result of this binding. Such binding followed by virolysis was demonstrated in Friend Murine Leukemia Virus (Rother et al. 1995), porcine endogenous retrovirus (PERV) (Takeuchi et al. 1996; Hayashi et al. 2004), HIV (Niel et al. 2005), pseudo-rabies virus, rhabdo-, lenti-, and spumaviruses (Takeuchi et al. 1997), Newcastle disease virus, Sindbis virus and vesicular stomatitis virus (Welsh et al. 1998; Pipperger et al. 2020), measles virus (Preece et al. 2002; Dürrbach et al. 2007) and vaccinia virus (Kim et al.). In all these examples, the viruses replicated in cells containing active α1,3GT, whereas replication of these viruses in human cells lacking α1,3GT resulted in no binding of human anti-Gal and no virolysis following incubation in human serum.

- *Targeting to APC by human anti-Gal* – The similarity between the GT-KO mouse and human anti-Gal can be further demonstrated by their ability to target anti-Gal immunocomplexed vaccines to APC, such as dendritic cells and macrophages via Fc/Fc receptor interaction. The ability of mouse anti-Gal to mediate such extensive uptake by opsonization was demonstrated above in the studies on OVA-liposomes vaccine (Figure 4). Such targeting was further visualized by the extensive uptake by mouse macrophages of rabbit RBC immunocomplexed with mouse anti-Gal, and no uptake without anti-Gal (LaTemple et al. 1999). The ability of human anti-Gal to opsonize particles and thus perform targeting to APC could be visualized with freshly obtained human lymphoma cells that were glycoengineered to present α-gal epitopes (as in Figure 1). The autologous anti-Gal of the studied patient bound to the glycoengineered lymphoma cells but not to the original lymphoma cells lacking α-gal epitope (Manches et al. 2005). Incubation for 2 hours at 37°C of the original and of glycoengineered lymphoma cells with autologous anti-Gal and with the APC of the patient resulted in extensive uptake of the tumor cells by macrophages and to a lesser extent into dendritic cells, whereas no such uptake was observed with the original lymphoma cells lacking α-gal epitopes (Figure 17). This uptake was inhibited in the presence of anti-CD64 antibody but not by anti-CD32 or anti-CD16 antibodies, implying that the uptake is mediate by high affinity FcγI receptors (Manches et al. 2005) which are present also on dendritic cells (Fanger et al. 1996).

All these studies strongly suggest that human anti-Gal and GT-KO mouse anti-Gal display great similarity in their characteristics, including their ability to form immune complexes with vaccinating viruses or virus envelope glycoproteins that are glycoengineered to present multiple α-gal epitopes. Thus, use of α-gal viral vaccines may be further evaluated in studies on safety and efficacy in primate and human trials.

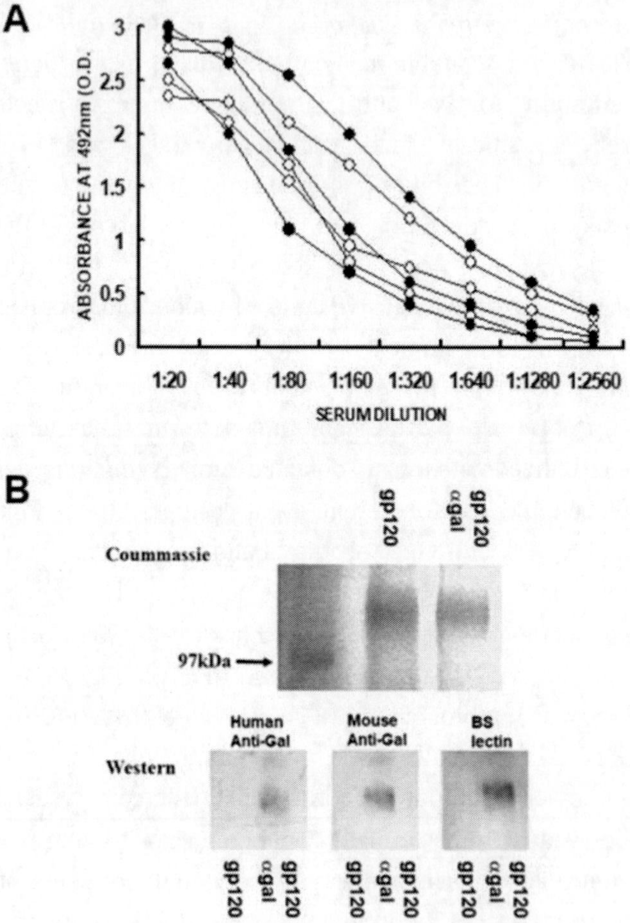

Figure 16. Similarities in activity of GT-KO mouse and human anti-Gal antibodies. A. Comparison of anti-Gal IgG activity in human sera (●) and sera of mice immunized with pig kidney membrane homogenate (O). Data are of 3 out of 30 humans and 30 GT-KO mice with similar results. B. Similarity in binding of both antibodies to *do novo* synthesized α-gal epitopes on gp120 by recombinant α1,3GT. The glycoproteins were subjected to SDS-PAGE electrophoresis followed and Western blotting. Upper gel: Coomassie staining of SDS-PAGE gel. Lower gels: Western blot stained with human anti-Gal, mouse anti-Gal, and the α-gal epitope specific *Bandeiraea simplicifolia* IB4 (BS) lectin. Note that the antibodies and the lectin bind to $gp120_{\alpha gal}$ and not to gp120. Modified from (Abdel-Motal et al. 2006).

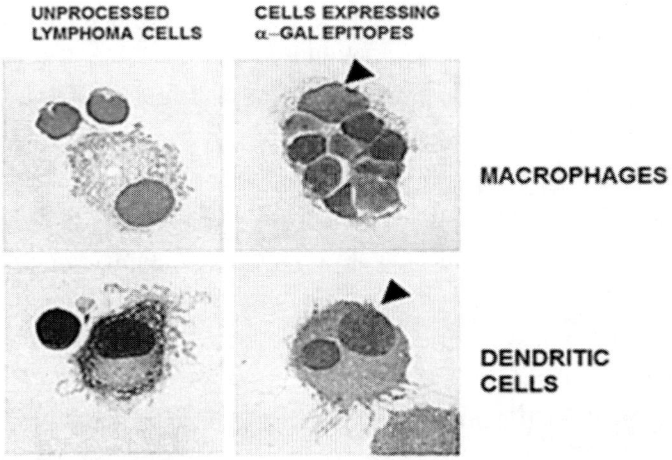

Figure 17. *In vitro* demonstration of anti-Gal mediated uptake of human B lymphoma cells by autologous APC. Human fresh lymphoma cells (B cell lymphoma) were subjected to the reactions in Figure 1 for the synthesis of α-Gal epitopes on the cell surface glycans. Lymphoma cells presenting α-gal epitopes or lacking them (i.e., original cells) were incubated with autologous anti-Gal for 30 min and subsequently, for 2 hours at 37°C with autologous macrophages or dendritic cells. At the end of incubation, the cells were placed on slides and stained. Arrowheads mark nuclei of the APC. Note the uptake of multiple glycoengineered lymphoma cells by the representative macrophage and of one lymphoma cell by the dendritic cell. No uptake of original lymphoma cells lacking α-gal epitopes was observed (x1000). Modified from (Manches et al. 2005).

METHODS FOR INCREASING EFFICACY OF COVID 19 VACCINES BY THEIR ANTI-GAL MEDIATED TARGETING TO APC

While writing this chapter, the world has been coping for 10 months with the Covid 19 pandemic with >35 million known infected individuals and an estimate of >1 million deaths associated with Covid 19 infection. There is an extensive effort for development of prophylactic vaccines against SARS-CoV-2 virus which causes the Covid 19 pandemic. As discussed below, there is a theoretical possibility that presently developed vaccines may be suboptimal for inducing immune protection against SARS-

CoV-2 in many elderly individuals. This section discusses possible reasons for suboptimal future vaccine immunogenicity among the elderly and describes methods for converting Covid 19 vaccines into α-gal vaccines, thereby amplifying their immunogenicity.

SARS-CoV-2 is an enveloped, single-stranded, positive-sense RNA virus that belongs to the Coronaviridae family (Zhou et al. 2020.) . The main target for vaccine development against SARS-CoV-2 infection is considered to be the spike (S) protein which is the major envelope glycoprotein of the virus. The notion that S protein may serve as a vaccine has been supported by studies demonstrating both neutralizing anti-S protein antibodies (Cao et al. 2020; Ju et. 2020) and memory T cells specific for the S protein in sera of convalescent COVID-19 patients (Grifoni et al. 2020; Ni et al. 2020). The S protein is present on the virus envelope as a trimer transmembrane protein that mediates attachment of SARS-CoV-2 to cells, fusion and entry into host cells (Wrapp et al. 2020). The S protein monomer is of the size of ~180 kDa and contains ~1300aa comprised of two functional subunits. The S1 subunit (~700 aa) mediates viral attachment to its cell surface "docking" receptor, the angiotensin converting enzyme 2 (ACE-2), and the S2 subunit (~600 aa) enables fusion of the virus with the cell membrane and penetration of the virus into the infected cell (Li et al. 2003; Letko et al. 2020; Wan et al. 2020). The S protein is has 22 N-glycans forming the glycan shied of SARS-CoV-2. Several of these glycans are of the high mannose type and the rest are of the complex type, as the left glycan in Figure 1.

The two main types of vaccines being developed against Covid 19 are: 1. Vaccines prepared of virus replicating in cell lines, including attenuated viruses, inactivated viruses, split vaccines, subunit vaccines prepared of the virus replicating in cell lines or produced as a recombinant protein in various expression systems, and virus-like particles. 2. Gene based vaccines prepared of nucleic acid (DNA or mRNA) containing the S protein gene. These gene based vaccines introduce the S protein gene into cells of the vaccinated individual and the transfected cells produce the vaccinating S protein which induces the generation of a protective immune response against the virus. The methods discussed in this section for increasing immunogenicity of S protein or of the whole SARS-CoV-2 virus, can be used only with the vaccines generated in the first group. The reason for this limitation is that glycoproteins produced in the vaccinated individual cannot be glycoengineered by the methods discussed below. In contrast, the inactivated whole virus, or the S protein as a subunit vaccine or as a recombinant protein are amenable to glycoengineering of the glycan shield, for converting glycans capped by sialic acid (left chain in Figure 1) into those presenting α-gal epitopes (right chain in Figure 1).

Initial clinical trials with gene base vaccines of SARS-CoV-2 S protein suggest that one vaccine injection does not suffice for inducing significant neutralizing antibody production in vaccinated individuals (Pedro et al. 2020; Jackson et al. 2020). A relatively low immunogenicity may be suggested by the great variability and modest levels of anti-S protein antibody production, observed in Covid 19 patients studied for post symptom detection onset (Xiao et al. 2020; Luchsinger et al. 2020). Taken together with the much higher proportion of elderly patients infected by and dying of Covid 19 compared to young patients (Cobos-Siles et al. 2020; Xie et al. 2020), it is possible that S protein vaccines may require amplification of their immunogenicity in order to increase the range of vaccinated individual benefiting from Covid 19 vaccines. Moreover, the need for providing Covid 19 vaccines worldwide to billions of individuals may require generation of vaccines that elicit a protective immune response with relatively low amounts of vaccinating material, i.e., vaccines with high immunogenicity.

As suggested in the Introduction section, the glycan shield of S protein is likely to negatively affect the immunogenicity of this glycoprotein. Two of the reasons for the low immunogenicity are: 1. The multiple sialic acid units on the glycans on the S protein generate an electrostatic negative charge that surrounds this glycoprotein and thus is likely to induce electrostatic repulsion with the sialic acid units on APC cell membrane glycans. This repulsion decreases the amount of vaccinating S protein molecules internalized by the APC due to random pinocytosis (Figure 2A). 2. The multiple glycans "camouflage" many of the immunogenic peptides of the S protein as they cover ~65% of S protein surface (Walls et al. 2016; Yang et al. 2020; Watanabe et al. 2020). This camouflage and the negative charge it generates further prevent many of the immunogenic peptides from engaging the corresponding B cell receptors in order to effectively activate B cells producing anti-S protein antibodies. The studies described in this chapter on the amplification of the immune response to influenza virus and to gp120 of HIV suggest that glycoengineering of the inactivated SARS-CoV-2 or of its S protein to present α-gal epitopes is likely to increase their immunogenicity, as well (Galili 2020b). In addition to the elimination of the negative electrostatic charges surrounding the S protein (Figure 2), anti-Gal will form immune complexes with the vaccinating inactivated SARS-CoV-$2_{\alpha gal}$ or with S protein $_{\alpha gal}$ and target these vaccines for effective uptake by APC via Fc/Fc receptor interaction (Figures 2B and 3). This extensive uptake of Covid 19 α-gal vaccines by APC will be followed by increased transport, processing and presentation of immunogenic S protein peptides within the lymph nodes, thereby increasing the probability of activation of the corresponding naive T and B cells in the elderly.

Glycoengineering of α-Gal Epitopes on Covid 19 Vaccines

Glycoengineering COVID 19 vaccines to present multiple α-gal epitopes may be achieved by a variety of methods. Some of these methods are described in this section:

1) *Neuraminidase and recombinant α1,3galactosyltransferase synthesizing α-gal epitopes on whole virus or on S protein* – The method for synthesis of α-gal epitopes on the inactivated SARS-CoV-2 or on subunit and recombinant S protein is illustrated in Figure 1. Neuraminidase, rα1,3GT and UDP-Gal are available from commercial sources. In the studies on the glycoengineering of influenza virus or of gp120, the rα1,3GT was produced by cloning truncated New World monkey (marmoset) α1,3GT cDNA lacking the cytoplasmic and transmembrane domains thereby allowing for secretion of the recombinant enzyme (Henion et al. 1994). The

enzyme also had a $(His)_6$ tag which enabled its purification. The production of rα1,3GT was performed in *Pichia pastoris* expression system stably transfected with this cDNA in a plasmid used for this expression system (Chen et al. 2001). The secreted enzyme was isolated by passing the medium through a nickel-Sepharose column which attaches the enzyme via a $(His)_6$ tag, followed by elution with imidazole. In addition to synthesis of multiple α-gal epitopes on influenza virus and on gp120, this rα1,3GT was found to effectively synthesize α-gal epitopes on human tumor cells by the two step enzymatic reaction illustrated in Figure 1 (Chen et al. 2001; Galili et al. 2003; Furukawa et al. 2017) and on a variety of mammalian RBC and nucleated cells (Ogawa & Galili, 2006). Thus, it is probable that inactivated SARS-CoV-2 or its S protein, subjected to the enzymatic reactions in Figure 1, will effectively undergo a similar conversion of the SA carrying glycan shield to multiple α-gal epitopes presented on the glycans. Whereas the resulting inactivated SARS-CoV-$2_{\alpha gal}$ can be isolated from the reaction mixture by precipitation or washing methods, the S $protein_{\alpha gal}$ can be purified by passing the reaction mixture through a column of the lectin *Bandeiraea simplicifolia* IB4 linked to Sepharose or to other porous beads. This lectin binds specifically α-gal epitopes (Wood et al. 1979), thus it would bind the S $protein_{\alpha gal}$ and no other components of the reaction mixture. The bound S $protein_{\alpha gal}$ may be eluted from the washed column by free galactose, melibiose or α-methyl galactoside, which subsequently may be removed by dialysis. It is not known whether chemical linking of α-gal epitope to the S protein (e.g., linking of the trisaccharide via a spacer to lysins) is a suitable method because such linking may affect the specificity of the immune response against the native protein.

2) *Syntheszing α-gal epitopes on replicating SARS-CoV-2 virus-* SARS-CoV-$2_{\alpha gal}$ is by engineering the host cells to effectively synthesized α-gal epitopes on the S protein of the virus envelope. As discussed above, complex type glycans on the S protein, as those

on other viral and cellular glycoproteins, are synthesize within compartments of the Golgi apparatus by a series of glycosyltransferases that add in a sequential manner carbohydrate units to the nascent carbohydrate chain on glycoproteins and glycolipids. Many of the glycans are "capped" with sialic acid which is linked to the glycan by sialyltransferases (SiaT), whereas the terminal galactose of the α-gal epitope is linked to the same glycan by α1,3GT. Both glycosyltransferases reside within the trans-Golgi compartment and compete with each other for capping the glycan (Smith et al. 1990). The ultimate number of α-gal epitopes vs. sialic acid epitopes on a virus depends on the relative activity of α1,3GT vs. that of SiaT. As shown in studies on activation of influenza virus specific T cells following anti-Gal mediated targeting of inactivated virus to APC, there is a correlation between the number of α-gal epitopes per vaccinating virus and the extent of T cell activation by peptides processed and presented by the APC (Galili et al. 1996). This suggests that by increasing the activity of α1,3GT within the trans-Golgi of host cells, more α-gal epitopes will be synthesized on the glycan shield of the replicating virus. Thus, it is possible that stable transfection of the host cell line in which SARS-CoV-2 is propagated, with several copies of the *α1,3GT* gene (*GGTA1*) will result increased activity of α1,3GT. A high number of copies of this gene will elevate the amount of α1,3GT thereby increasing the number of synthesized α-gal epitopes on the S protein of the replicating virus. This assumption is supported by studies demonstrating that measles virus replicating in human host cells transfected with the *α1,3GT* gene present α-gal epitopes binding anti-Gal on their envelope glycoproteins (Preece et al. 2002; Dürrbach et al. 2007). A similar effect of increased number of α-gal epitopes on the virus may be achieved by disruption (i.e., knockout) of SiaT genes in host cells which will result in decreased competition of SiaT capping the glycans with SA and α1,3GT thus, enabling α1,3GT capping more glycans with α-gal epitopes. Since part of the glycans on the S protein are of the high mannose type, it is further possible that by disrupting genes associated with synthesis of high mannose glycans, more glycans will be synthesized as complex type glycans which enable additional synthesis of α-gal epitopes. Thus, an optimal host cell for production of SARS-CoV-2 with multiple α-gal epitopes may be a cell with several copies of the *α1,3GT* gene, with reduced SiaT activity and possibly with reduced proportion of glycans of the high mannose type. It should be noted that the glycans on SARS-CoV-2 also may affect the extent of replication of the virus in the host cell. Thus, following each genetic manipulation step of the host cells, the extent of virus replication should be determined in order to confirm that it is was not affected. A similar approach may be considered for cell expression systems producing recombinant S protein and for cells producing SARS-CoV-2 virus like particles. All these vaccine materials may be produced with a large number of α-gal epitopes on the glycan shield in cells that have several copies of the α1,3GT gene, disrupted SiaT genes and possibly disrupted genes of enzymes synthesizing high mannose glycans.

3) *Transduction with replication defective adenovirus containing the α1,3GT gene for synthesis of α-gal epitopes on vaccinating viruses* – Multiple copies of the *α1,3GT* gene may be introduce into host cells also by transduction with replication defective adenovirus containing the *α1,3GT* gene (Deriy et al. 2002), prior to infection of the cells with SARS-CoV-2. Mouse α1,3GT cDNA was inserted into a replication-defective adenovirus vector which lacks the E1 and E2 genes (Gao et al. 1996). This viral vector, designated AdαGT, could be propagated in human 293 cells that have the viral E1 complementing gene. Transduction of human HeLa cells with AdαGT resulted in immediate penetration of ~20 AdαGT copies into each cell and the appearance of α1,3GT mRNA after 4 hours (Deriy et al. 2002). Analysis of the appearance of α1,3GT catalytic activity within the transduced cells at various time points

demonstrated activity of this enzyme 6 hours post transduction. The α-gal epitopes were first detected on the cell surface glycans 10 hours post transduction. After 24 hours, each cell expressed ~2 x 10^6 epitopes and after 48 hours the cells expressed a maximum number of 4 x 10^6 epitopes per cell. Thus, it is suggested that transduction of host cells with AdαGT 12-24 hours prior to the infection of the cells with SARS-CoV-2 may result in effective synthesis of α-gal epitopes on the replicating virus. Since the number of complex type glycans vs. that of high mannose glycans may vary from one cell line to the other, a cell line producing virus with the highest number of glycans of the complex type may be preferable for intracellular synthesis of α-gal epitopes on SARS-CoV-2. Alternatively, glycoengineering the optimal cell line for decrease or elimination of high mannose glycans may require the inactivation of gene(s) associated with synthesis of such glycans. Glycoengineering of cells producing the S protein by methods suggested above for host cells producing replicating virus with maximum α-gal epitopes may also be applicable the S protein producing cells.

4) *Production of S protein$_{\alpha gal}$ in glycoengineered yeasts*– Production of relatively large amounts of recombinant S protein$_{\alpha gal}$ may be achieved in yeast expression systems by stable transfection of the yeast cells with the S protein. However, in order to achieve synthesis of α-gal epitopes on the S protein product, yeast need to undergo additional glycoengineering manipulation since naturally, yeast have glycosyltransferases that can synthesize N-linked glycans only of the high mannose type. Glycoproteins which carry only the high mannose N-linked glycans have short half-life in humans. For production of glycoproteins with complex type glycans, yeasts such as *Pichia pastoris* have been glycoengineered to synthesize humanized glycans with the terminal structure of complex type by introducing the corresponding glycosyltransferase genes (Choi et al. 2003; Wildt & Gerngross, 2005). In order to produce S protein with glycan shield presenting multiple α-gal epitopes, the *SiaT* gene in

these yeasts may be replaced by the *α1,3GT* gene (*GGTA1*). It remains to be determined whether such a manipulation is feasible and to what extent this expression system can produce sufficiently large amounts of S protein$_{\alpha gal}$ for preparation of a high number of vaccines.

5) *Production of S protein$_{\alpha gal}$ in glycoengineered bacteria* – Bacteria such as *E. coli* may also be engineered to produce S protein$_{\alpha gal}$. Production of recombinant proteins in bacteria has been limited because of the difficulties in secretion of recombinant proteins beyond the periplasmic space into the culture medium. Secretion of such recombinant proteins has been achieved by the use of a nonionic detergent such as Triton X-100 (Fu, 2010). Secretion of a recombinant protein also could be achieved by modifying the protein for targeting it to the outer membrane and further into the extracellular medium (Fisher et al. 2011). Other studies have demonstrated biosynthesis of α-gal epitope oligosaccharides in *E. coli* by introducing into this bacterium genes coding for the sequence of mammalian glycosyltransferases including α1,3GT, required for α-gal epitope synthesis (Chen et al. 2000; Gebus et al. 2012). Moreover, *E. coli* was engineered to synthesize N-linked glycans by transfer into it an N-linked glycosylation system found in *Campylobacter jejuni* (Wacker et al. 2002; Fisher et al. 2011). It is suggested that combining these characteristics by introducing the genes coding for the above enzymes into one bacterial strain may lead to the production of an expression system that effectively produces S protein$_{\alpha gal}$ in quality and amounts suitable for vaccine preparation.

Potential Safety Issues with Future α-Gal Vaccines in Humans

Humans are regularly exposed to α-gal epitopes in meat such as beef, pork and lamb. However, relatively few individuals have been exposed to this epitope administered in the form of injection. This raises the question whether administration of vaccines presenting α-gal epitopes is safe in humans. The most common example of α-gal epitopes administration into humans in a form that is constantly exposed to the blood circulation is the replacement of impaired heart valves with bioprostheses of porcine heart valves or of bovine pericardium crosslinked by glutaraldehyde. Like other porcine and bovine tissues, these valves present multiple α-gal epitopes (Tanemura et al. 2000). No toxicity or other deleterious effects have been observed in association with this treatment which is widely used for replacement of impaired heart valves in elderly and young patients, respectively. Phase I clinical trials in which α-gal glycolipids are injected into solid tumors of cancer patients, in order to convert the tumor into autologous anti-tumor vaccines, also were found to be safe and demonstrated no adverse effects (Whalen et al. 2012; Albertini et al. 2016). Similarly, synthesis of α-gal epitopes on autologous tumor cell membranes followed by their incubation with anti-Gal and autologous dendritic cells, was performed for converting autologous tumors into vaccines. Injection of such mixtures into patients was reported to be safe with no adverse effects, as well (Qiu et al. 2011; 2013; 2016).

A small proportion of individuals in various populations was found to produce anti-Gal IgE antibodies following the bite of several kinds of ticks including *Ambliomma Americanum* (Lone Star tick) in USA (Commins & Platts-Mills, 2013), *Ixodes ricinus* in Europe (Hamsten et al. 2013), *Haemaphysalis longicornis* in Japan (Chinuki et al. 2016) and *Ixodes holocyclus* in Australia (van Nunen, 2015). This IgE mediates allergic response to α-gal epitopes in meat is referred to as "α-gal syndrome" (Wilson et al. 2017; Pollack et al. 2019). If viral vaccines presenting α-gal epitopes are developed for use in humans, it remains to be determined whether individuals with α-gal syndrome display adverse effects following administration of α-gal vaccine. In addition, vaccination of such individuals with α-gal vaccine will enable determining whether they require anti-allergy treatment prior to vaccination.

CONCLUSION

Production of the natural anti-Gal antibody in large amounts in all humans who are not severely immunocompromised, enables development of several novel immunotherapies. In these immunotherapies, the interaction between anti-Gal and the carbohydrate antigen it recognizes- the "α-gal epitope," may be applied for generating a variety of immune responses that can be beneficial to treated patients (Galili, 2013a; 2018). One of these applications is the amplification of viral vaccines efficacy by glycoengineering the glycan shield of glycoproteins on enveloped viruses to present multiple α-gal epitope and thus produce α-gal vaccines. Administration of viral α-gal vaccines in the form of inactivated whole virus vaccine, or of envelope glycoprotein vaccine results in formation of immune complexes with the natural anti-Gal antibody. This antibody is released from capillaries ruptured by the syringe needle at the vaccination site. The complement activation by such immune complexes results in generation of chemotactic peptides that recruit APC to the injected vaccine suspension or solution. This is followed by extensive endocytosis of the vaccine/anti-Gal immune complexes into the APC, instead of random suboptimal uptake by pinocytosis of standard non-immunocomplexed vaccines. The endocytosis is induced by interaction between the Fc portion of immunocomplexed anti-Gal and Fc receptors on APC and possibly between C3b attached to the immune complexes and C3b receptors (CR1) on APC. The internalized vaccines are processed within the APC and their immunogenic peptides are presented on cell surface MHC molecules. Transport of these vaccines by APC to regional lymph nodes results in activation of many virus specific helper and cytotoxic T cells which may effectively prevent the subsequent detrimental infection by the corresponding infectious virus. Studies in anti-Gal producing mice on the efficacy of α-gal vaccines, including inactivated whole influenza virus and recombinant gp120 of HIV, demonstrated 10-200 fold increase in the immune response with α-gal vaccines vs. vaccine lacking α-gal epitopes. Studies of challenge with a lethal dose of infectious influenza virus demonstrated 8 fold higher resistance to challenge of a lethal infection dose in mice immunized with α-gal vaccine than in the absence of α-gal epitopes on the vaccine. The α-gal vaccine method can further enable increasing immunity of internal viral proteins of low immunity by formation of fusion α-gal vaccines between virus envelope glycoprotetin and virus internal protein such as $gp120_{\alpha gal}/p24$ of HIV which was found to greatly increase immunogenicity of both gp120 and p24.

The studies of influenza virus and gp120 α-gal vaccines strongly suggest that glycoengineering of SARS-CoV-2 inactivated whole virus and of this virus envelope S protein vaccines to present α-gal epitopes will markedly increase the immunogenicity and efficacy of these Covid-19 vaccines. This is because the number of N-linked glycans on the S protein is high, thereby ensuring the synthesis of many α-gal epitopes on the glycan shield of this envelope glycoprotein. Synthesis of multiple α-gal epitopes on SARS-CoV-2 or on S protein vaccines may be feasible by several methods. These include: *In vitro* enzymatic synthesis; propagating the virus in host cells engineered to contain many copies of the *α1,3GT* gene (*GGTA1*) by stable transfection; transduction of host cells with replication defective AdαGT virus; production of S $protein_{\alpha gal}$ in mammalian cell, yeast, or bacterial expression systems engineered to contain the glycosyltransferase transgenes required for the synthesis of α-gal epitopes.

Introduction of α-gal epitopes into humans, on glycans porcine heart valve or as glycolipids in cancer immunotherapy suggest that α-gal vaccines may be safe in humans. However, since a small proportion of humans display delayed allergic response to α-gal epitopes in meat ("α-gal syndrome"), it should be determined whether individuals with α-gal syndrome require anti-allergy treatment prior to receiving α-gal vaccines.

References

Abdel-Motal U, Wang S, Lu S, Wigglesworth K, Galili U. Increased immunogenicity of human immunodeficiency virus gp120 engineered to express Galα1-3Galβ1-4GlcNAc-R epitopes. *J Virol* 2006; 80: 6943-51.

Abdel-Motal UM, Guay HM, Wigglesworth K, Welsh RM, Galili U. Immunogenicity of influenza virus vaccine is increased by anti-Gal-mediated targeting to antigen-presenting cells. *J Virol* 2007; 81: 9131-41.

Abdel-Motal UM, Wigglesworth K, Galili U. Intratumoral injection of α-gal glycolipids induces a protective anti-tumor T cell response which overcomes Treg activity. *Cancer Immunol Immunother* 2009a; 58: 1545-56.

Abdel-Motal UM, Wigglesworth K, Galili U. Mechanism for increased immunogenicity of vaccines that form in vivo immune complexes with the natural anti-Gal antibody. *Vaccine* 2009b; 27: 3072-82.

Abdel-Motal UM, Wang S, Awad A, Lu S, Wigglesworth K, Galili U. Increased immunogenicity of HIV-1 p24 and gp120 following immunization with gp120/p24 fusion protein vaccine expressing α-gal epitopes. *Vaccine* 2010; 28: 1758-65.

Ahlén G, Frelin L. Methods to evaluate novel hepatitis C virus vaccines. *Methods Mol Biol* 2016; 1403: 221-44.

Akbar AN, Gilroy DW. Aging immunity may exacerbate COVID-19. *Science* 2020; 369: 256-57.

Albertini MR, Ranheim EA, Zuleger CL, Sondel PM, Hank JA, Bridges A, et al. Phase I study to evaluate toxicity and feasibility of intratumoral injection of α-gal glycolipids in patients with advanced melanoma. *Cancer Immunol Immunother* 2016; 65: 897-907.

Ambrozaitis A, Groth N, Bugarini R, Sparacio V, Podda A, Lattanzi M. A novel mammalian cell-culture technique for consistent production of a well tolerated and immunogenic trivalent subunit influenza vaccine. *Vaccine* 2009; 27: 6022-29.

Banchereau J, Steinman RM. Dendritic cells and the control of immunity. *Nature* 1998; 392: 245-52.

Basu M, Basu S. Enzymatic synthesis of blood group related pentaglycosyl ceramide by an α-galactosyltransferase. *J Biol Chem* 1973; 248: 1700-6.

Benatuil L, Kaye J, Rich RF, Fishman JA, Green WR, Iacomini J. The influence of natural antibody specificity on antigen immunogenicity. *Eur J Immunol* 2005; 35: 2638-47.

Berzofsky JA, Ahlers JD, Janik, J. Morris J, Oh S, Terabe M, et al. Progress on new vaccine strategies against chronic viral infections. *J Clin Invest* 2004; 114: 450-62.

Blake DA, Goldstein IJ. An α-D-galactosyltransferase activity in Ehrlich ascites tumor cells. Biosynthesis and characterization of a trisaccharide (α-D-galactose-(1-3)-N-acetyllactosamine). *J Biol Chem* 1981; 256: 5387-93.

Blanken WM, Van den Eijnden DH. Biosynthesis of terminal Galα1-3Galβ1-4GlcNAc-R oligosaccharide sequences on glycoconjugates. Purification and acceptor specificity of a UDP-Gal:N-acetyllactosaminide α1-3-galactosyltransferase from calf thymus. *J Biol Chem* 1985; 260: 12927-34.

Blixt O, Head S, Mondala T, Scanlan C, Huflejt ME, Alvarez R, et al. Printed covalent glycan array for ligand profiling of diverse glycan binding proteins. *Proc Natl Acad Sci USA* 2004; 101: 17033-38.

Bovin N. Natural antibodies to glycans. *Biochemistry (Moscow)* 2013; 78: 786-97.

Cao Y, Su B, Guo X, Sun W, Deng Y, Bao L, et al. Potent neutralizing antibodies against SARS-CoV-2 identified by high-throughput single-cell sequencing of convalescent patients' B cells. *Cell* 2020; 182: 73-84.

CDC COVID-19 Response Team. Severe Outcomes Among Patients with Coronavirus Disease 2019 (COVID-19) - United States, February 12-March 16, 2020. *MMWR Morb Mortal Wkly Rep* 2020; 69: 343-46.

Celis E, Chang TW. Antibodies to hepatitis B surface antigen potentiate the response of human T lymphocyte clones to the same antigen. *Science* 1984; 224: 297-9.

Chang YT, Guo CY, Tsai MS, Cheng YY, Lin MT, Chen CH, et al. Poor immune response to a standard single dose non-adjuvanted vaccination against 2009 pandemic H1N1 influenza virus A in the adult and elder hemodialysis patients. *Vaccine* 2012; 30: 5009-18.

Chen X, Liu Z, Wang J, Fang J, Fan H, Wang PG. Changing the donor cofactor of bovine α1,3-galactosyltransferase by fusion with UDP-galactose 4- epimerase. More efficient biocatalysis for synthesis of α-Gal epitopes. *J Biol Chem* 2000; 275: 31594-600.

Chen ZC, Tanemura M, Galili U. Synthesis of α-gal epitopes (Galα1-3Galβ1-4GlcNAc-R) on human tumor cells by recombinant α1,3galactosyltransferase produced in *Pichia pastoris*. *Glycobiology* 2001; 11: 577-86.

Chinuki Y, Ishiwata K, Yamaji K, Takahashi H, Morita E. *Haemaphysalis longicornis* tick bites are a possible cause of red meat allergy in Japan. *Allergy* 2016; 71: 421-5.

Choi BK, Bobrowicz P, Davidson RC, Hamilton SR, Kung DH, Li H, et al. Use of combinatorial genetic libraries to humanize N-linked glycosylation in the yeast *Pichia pastoris*. *Proc Natl Acad Sci USA* 2003; 100: 5022-27.

Clynes R, Takechi Y, Moroi Y, Houghton A, Ravetch JV. Fc receptors are required in passive and active immunity to melanoma. *Proc Natl Acad Sci USA* 1998; 95: 652-56.

Cobos-Siles M, Cubero-Morais P, Arroyo-Jiménez I, et al. Cause-specific death in hospitalized individuals infected with SARS-CoV-2: more than just acute respiratory failure or thromboembolic events (published online ahead of print, 2020 Sep 10). *Intern Emerg Med* 2020; 10.1007/s11739-020-02485-y.

Commins SP, Platts-Mills TA. Tick bites and red meat allergy. *Curr Opin Allergy Clin Immunol* 2013; 13: 354-9.

Cooper DKC, Good AH, Koren E, Oriol R, Malcolm AJ, Ippolito RM, et al. Identification of α-galactosyl and other carbohydrate epitopes that are bound by human anti-pig antibodies: Relevance to discordant xenografting in man. *Transpl Immunol* 1993; 1: 198-205.

Couch RB, Keitel WA, Cate TR. Improvement of inactivated influenza virus vaccines. *J Infect Dis* 1997; 176: Suppl 1, S38-44.

Crooks E, Tong T, Chakrabarti B, Narayan K, Georgiev I, Menis, S. Vaccine-elicited Tier 2 HIV-1 neutralizing antibodies bind to quaternary epitopes involving glycan-deficient patches proximal to the CD4 binding site. *PLoS Pathog* 2015; 11: e1004932.

Deriy L, Chen ZC, Gao GP, Galili U. Expression of α-gal epitopes on HeLa cells transduced with adenovirus containing α1,3galactosyltransferase cDNA. *Glycobiology* 2002; 12: 135-44.

Dor FJM, Tseng YL, Cheng J, Moran K, Sanderson TM, Lancos CJ, et al. α1,3-Galactosyltransferase gene-knockout miniature swine produce natural cytotoxic anti-Gal antibodies. *Transplantation* 2004; 78: 15-20.

Dürrbach A, Baple E, Preece AF, Charpentier B, Gustafsson K. Virus recognition by specific natural antibodies and complement results in MHC I cross-presentation. *J Immunol* 2007; 37: 1254-65.

Estrada LD, Schultz-Cherry S. Development of a universal influenza vaccine. *J Immunol* 2019; 202: 392-98.

Fang J, Walters A, Hara H, Long C, Yeh P, Ayares D, et al. Anti-gal antibodies in α1,3-galactosyltransferase gene-knockout pigs. *Xenotransplantation* 2012; 19: 305-310.

Fanger NA, Wardwell K, Shen L, Tedder TF, Guyre PM. Type I (CD64) and type II (CD32) Fc gamma receptor-mediated phagocytosis by human blood dendritic cells. *J Immunol* 1996; 157: 541-8.

Fiers W, De Filette M, Birkett A, Neirynck S, Min Jou W. A ''universal" human influenza A vaccine. *Virus Res* 2004;103:173-76.

Fisher AC, Haitjema CH, Guarino C, Çelik E, Endicott CE, Reading CA, et al. Production of secretory and extracellular N-linked glycoproteins in *Escherichia coli*. *Appl Environ Microbiol* 2011; 77: 871-81.

Fu XY. Extracellular accumulation of recombinant protein by *Escherichia coli* in a defined medium. *Appl Microbiol Biotechnol* 2010; 88: 75-86.

Furukawa K, Tanemura M, Miyoshi E, Eguchi H, Nagano H, Matsunami K, et al. A practical approach to pancreatic cancer immunotherapy using resected tumor lysate vaccines processed to express α-gal epitopes. *PLoS One* 2017; 12: e0184901.

Galili U. Interaction of the natural anti-Gal antibody with α-galactosyl epitopes: A major obstacle for xenotransplantation in humans. *Immunol. Today* 1993; 14: 480-482.

Galili U. Anti-Gal: an abundant human natural antibody of multiple pathogeneses and clinical benefits. *Immunology* 2013a; 140: 1-11.

Galili U. α1,3Galactosyltransferase knockout pigs produce the natural anti-Gal antibody and simulate the evolutionary appearance of this antibody in primates. *Xenotransplantation* 2013b; 20: 267-76.

Galili U. *The natural anti-Gal antibody as foe turned friend in medicine.* Academic Press/Elsevier, Publishers, London (2018).

Galili U. Evolution in primates by "Catastrophic-selection" interplay between enveloped virus epidemics, mutated genes of enzymes synthesizing carbohydrate antigens, and natural anti-carbohydrate antibodies. *Am J Phys Anthropol* 2019; 168: 352-63.

Galili U. Human natural antibodies to mammalian carbohydrate antigens as unsung heroes protecting against past, present, and future viral infections. *Antibodies* (Basel). 2020a; 9(2): 25.

Galili U. Amplifying immunogenicity of prospective Covid-19 vaccines by glycoengineering the coronavirus glycan-shield to present α-gal epitopes. *Vaccine* 2020b; 38: 6487-99.

Galili U, Rachmilewitz EA, Peleg A, Flechner I. A unique natural human IgG antibody with anti-α-galactosyl specificity. *J Exp Med* 1984; 160: 1519-31.

Galili U, Macher BA, Buehler J, Shohet SB. Human natural anti-α-galactosyl IgG. II. The specific recognition of α(1,3)-linked galactose residues. *J Exp Med* 1985; 162: 573-82.

Galili U, Buehler J, Shohet SB, Macher BA. The human natural anti-Gal IgG. III. The subtlety of immune tolerance in man as demonstrated by crossreactivity between natural anti-Gal and anti-B antibodies. *J Exp Med* 1987a; 165: 693-704.

Galili U, Clark MR, Shohet SB, Buehler J, Macher BA. Evolutionary relationship between the anti-Gal antibody and the Galα1-3Gal epitope in primates. *Proc Natl Acad Sci USA* 1987b; 84: 1369-73.

Galili U, Mandrell RE, Hamadeh RM, Shohet SB, Griffiss JM. Interaction between human natural anti-α-galactosyl immunoglobulin G and bacteria of the human flora. *Infect Immun* 1988a; 56: 1730-37.

Galili U, Shohet SB, Kobrin E, Stults CLM, Macher BA. Man, apes, and Old World monkeys differ from other mammals in the expression of α-galactosyl epitopes on nucleated cells. *J Biol Chem* 1988b; 263: 17755-62.

Galili U, Swanson K. Gene sequences suggest inactivation of α-1,3-galactosyltransferase in catarrhines after the divergence of apes from monkeys. *Proc Natl Acad Sci USA* 1991; 88: 7401-4.

Galili U, Anaraki F, Thall A, Hill-Black C, Radic M. One percent of circulating B lymphocytes are capable of producing the natural anti-Gal antibody. *Blood* 1993; 82: 2485-93.

Galili U, LaTemple DC. Natural anti-Gal antibody as a universal augmenter of autologous tumor vaccine immunogenicity. *Immunol Today* 1997; 18: 281-85.

Galili U, Repik PM, Anaraki F, Mozdzanowska K, Washko G, Gerhard W. Enhancement of antigen presentation of influenza virus hemagglutinin by the natural human anti-Gal antibody. *Vaccine* 1996; 14: 321-28.

Galili U, LaTemple DC, Radic MZ. A sensitive assay for measuring α-gal epitope expression on cells by a monoclonal anti-Gal antibody. *Transplantation* 1998; 65: 1129-32.

Galili U, Chen ZC, DeGeest K. Expression of α-gal epitopes on ovarian carcinoma membranes to be used as a novel autologous tumor vaccine. *Gynecol Oncol* 2003; 90: 100-8.

Galili U, Wigglesworth K, Abdel-Motal UM. Intratumoral injection of α-gal glycolipids induces xenograft-like destruction and conversion of lesions into endogenous vaccines. *J Immunol* 2007; 178: 4676-87.

Gao GP, Yang Y, Wilson JM. Biology of adenovirus vectors with E1 and E4 deletions for liver-directed gene therapy. *J Virol* 1996; 70: 8934-43.

Gebus C, Cottin C, Randriantsoa M, Drouillard S, Samain E. Synthesis of αgalactosyl epitopes by metabolically engineered *Escherichia coli*. *Carbohydr Res* 2012; 361: 83-90.

Geyer H, Holschbach C, Hunsmann G, Schneider J. Carbohydrates of human immunodeficiency virus. Structures of oligosaccharides linked to the envelope glycoprotein 120. *J Biol Chem* 1988; 263: 11760-67.

Good AH, Cooper DCK, Malcolm AJ, Ippolito RM, Koren E, Neethling FA, et al. Identification of carbohydrate structures which bind human anti-porcine antibodies: Implication for discordant xenografting in man. *Transplant Proc* 1992; 24: 559-62.

Gosselin EJ, Wardwell K, Gosselin DR, Alter N, Fisher JL, Guyre PM. Enhanced antigen presentation using human Fc gamma receptor (monocyte/macrophage)-specific immunogens. *J Immunol* 1992; 149: 3477-81.

Goulder PJ, Watkins DI. HIV and SIV CTL escape: implications for vaccine design. *Nat Rev Immunol* 2004; 4: 630-40.

Grifoni A, Weiskopf D, Ramirez SI, Mateus J, Dan JM, Moderbacher CR, et al. Targets of T Cell rresponses to SARS-CoV-2 Coronavirus in humans with COVID-19 disease and unexposed individuals. *Cell* 2020; 181: 1489-1501.

Hamadeh RM, Galili U, Zhou P, Griffiss JM. Human secretions contain IgA, IgG and IgM anti-Gal (anti-α-galactosyl) antibodies. *Clin Diagn Lab Immunol* 1995; 2: 125-31.

Hamsten C, Starkhammar M, Tran TA, Johansson M, Bengtsson U, Ahlén G, et al. Identification of galactose-α-1,3-galactose in the gastrointestinal tract of the tick *Ixodes ricinus*; possible relationship with red meat allergy. *Allergy* 2013; 68: 549-52.

Hayashi S, Ogawa S, Takashima Y, Otsuka H. The neutralization of pseudorabies virus by anti-α-galactosyl natural antibody in normal serum. *Virus Res* 2004; 99: 1-7.

Henion TR, Macher BA, Anaraki F, Galili U. Defining the minimal size of catalytically active primate α1,3galactosyltransferase: structure-function studies on the recombinant truncated enzyme. *Glycobiology* 1994; 4: 193-201.

Henion TR, Gerhard W, Anaraki F, Galili U. Synthesis of α-gal epitopes on influenza virus vaccines by recombinant α1,3galactosyltransferase enables the formation of immune complexes with the natural anti-Gal antibody. *Vaccine* 1997; 15: 1174-82.

Hooperm LV, Macpherson AJ. Immune adaptations that maintain homeostasis with intestinal microbiota. *Nat Rev Immunol* 2010; 10: 159-69.

Houston WE, Kremer RJ, Crabbs CL, Spertzel RO. Inactivated Venezuelan equine encephalomyelitis virus vaccine complexed with specific antibody: enhanced primary immune response and altered pattern of antibody class elicited. *J Infect Dis* 1977; 135: 600-10.

Iniguez E, Schocker NS, Subramaniam K, Portillo S, Montoya AL, Al-Salem WS, et al. An α-Gal-containing neoglycoprotein-based vaccine partially protects against murine cutaneous leishmaniasis caused by *Leishmania major*. *PLoS Negl Trop Dis* 2017; 11: e0006039.

Iuliano AD, Roguski KM, Chang HH, Muscatello DJ, Palekar R, Tempia S, et al. Estimates of global seasonal influenza-associated respiratory mortality: a modelling study. *Lancet* 2018; 391: 1285-1300.

Jackson LA, Anderson EJ, Rouphael NG, Roberts PC, Makhene M, Coler RN, et al. An mRNA Vaccine against SARS-CoV-2 — Preliminary Report. *N Engl J Med* 2020: DOI: 10.1056/NEJMoa2022483.

Ju B, Zhang Q, Ge J, Wang R, Sun J, Ge X, Yu J, et al. Human neutralizing antibodies elicited by SARS-CoV-2 infection. *Nature* 2020; 584: 115-19.

Katz JM, Plowden J, Renshaw-Hoelscher M, Lu X, Tumpey TM, Sambhara S. Immunity to influenza: the challenges of protecting an aging population. *Immunol Res* 2004; 29: 113-24.

Kendall MD, Johnson HR, Singh J. The weight of the human thymus gland at necropsy. *J Anat* 1980; 131: 483-97.

Keil W, Geyer R, Dabrowski J, Dabrowski U, Niemann H, Stirm S, et al. Carbohydrates of influenza virus. Structural elucidation of the individual glycans of the FPV hemagglutinin by two-dimensional 1H n.m.r. and methylation analysis. *EMBO J* 1985; 4: 2711-20.

Kim NY, Jung WW, Oh YK, Chun T, Park HY, Lee HT, et al. Natural protection from zoonosis by α-gal epitopes on virus particles in xenotransmission. *Xenotransplantation* 2007; 14: 104-11.

Kiyono H, Kunisawa J, McGhee JR, Mestecky J. The Mucosal Immune System. In: Paul, WE., editor. *Fundamental Immunology.* Lippincott Williams & Wilkins; Philadelphia, PA, 2008; pp. 983-1030.

Koike C, Fung JJ, Geller DA, Kannagi R, Libert T, Luppi P, et al. Molecular basis of evolutionary loss of the α1,3-galactosyltransferase gene in higher primates. *J Biol Chem* 2002; 277: 10114-20.

Lai L, Kolber-Simonds D, Park KW, Cheong HT, Greenstein JL, Im GS, et al. Production of α-1,3-galactosyltransferase knockout pigs by nuclear transfer cloning. *Science* 2002; 295: 1089-92.

Lanteri M, Giordanengo V, Vidal F, Gaudray P, Lefebvre JC. A complete α1,3-galactosyltransferase gene is present in the human genome and partially transcribed. *Glycobiology* 2002; 12: 785-92.

Larsen RD, Rivera-Marrero CA, Ernst LK, Cummings RD, Lowe JB. Frameshift and nonsense mutations in a human genomic sequence homologous to a murine UDP-Gal:β-D-Gal(1,4)-D-GlcNAc α(1,3)-galactosyltransferase cDNA. *J Biol Chem* 1990; 265: 7055-61.

LaTemple DC, Abrams JT, Zhang, Galili U. Increased immunogenicity of tumor vaccines complexed with anti-Gal: Studies in knock out mice for α1,3galactosyltranferase. *Cancer Res* 1999; 59: 3417-23.

Leonard CK, Spellman MW, Riddle L, Harris RJ, Thomas JN, Gregory TJ. Assignment of intrachain disulfide bonds and characterization of potential glycosylation sites of the type 1 recombinant human immunodeficiency virus envelope glycoprotein (gp120) expressed in Chinese hamster ovary cells. *J Biol Chem* 1990; 265: 10373-82.

Letko M, Marzi A, Munster V. Functional assessment of cell entry and receptor usage for SARS-CoV-2 and other lineage B betacoronaviruses. *Nat Microbiol* 2020; 5: 562-69.

Letvin NL. Progress toward an HIV vaccine. *Annu Rev Med* 2005; 56: 213-23.

Lewis GK, DeVico AL, Gallo RC. Antibody persistence and T-cell balance: two key factors confronting HIV vaccine development. *Proc Natl Acad Sci USA* 2014; 111: 15614-21.

Li W, Moore MJ, Vasilieva N, Sui J, Wong SW, Berne MA, et al. Angiotensin-converting enzyme 2 is a functional receptor for the SARS coronavirus. *Nature* 2003; 426: 450-54.

Liu K, Chen Y, Lin R, Han K. Clinical features of COVID-19 in elderly patients: A comparison with young and middle-aged patients. *J Infect* 2020; 2020; 80: e14-e18.

Luchsinger LL, Ransegnola B, Jin D, Muecksch F, Weisblum Y, Bao W, et al. Serological assays estimate highly variable SARS-CoV-2 neutralizing antibody activity in recovered COVID19 patients (published online ahead of print, 2020 Sep 11). *J Clin Microbiol* 2020; JCM.02005-20.

Manca F, Fenoglio D, Li Pira G, Kunkl A, Celada F. Effect of antigen/antibody ratio on macrophage uptake, processing, and presentation to T cells of antigen complexed with polyclonal antibodies. *J Exp Med* 1991; 173: 37-48.

Manches O, Plumas J, Lui G, Chaperot L, Molens J-P, Sotto J-J, et al. Anti-Gal-mediated targeting of human B lymphoma cells to antigen-presenting cells: a potential method for immunotherapy using autologous tumor cells. *Haematologica* 2005; 90: 625-34.

Mañez R, Blanco FJ, Díaz I, Centeno A, Lopez-Pelaez E, Hermida M, et al. Removal of bowel aerobic gram-negative bacteria is more effective than immunosuppression with cyclophosphamide and steroids to decrease natural α-galactosyl IgG antibodies. *Xenotransplantation* 2001; 8: 15-23.

Matsumoto A, Yoshima H, Kobata A. Carbohydrates of influenza virus hemagglutinin: structures of the whole neutral sugar chains. *Biochemistry* 1983; 22: 188-96.

McMorrow IM, Comrack CA, Sachs DH, DerSimonian H. Heterogeneity of human anti-pig natural antibodies cross-reactive with the Gal(α1,3)Galactose epitope. *Transplantation* 1997, 64, 501-510.

Mizuochi T, Matthews T, Kato M, Hamako J, Titani K, Solomon J, et al. Diversity of oligosaccharide structures on the envelope glycoprotein gp120 of human immunodeficiency virus 1 from the lymphoblastoid cell line H9. Presence of complex-type oligosaccharides with bisecting N-acetylglucosamine residues. *J Biol Chem* 1990; 265: 8519-24.

Montefiori DC, Pantaleo G, Fink LM, Zhou JT, Zhou JY, Bilska M, et al. Neutralizing and infection-enhancing antibody responses to human immunodeficiency virus type 1 in long-term nonprogressors. *J Infect Dis* 1996; 173: 60-77.

Munier CM, Andersen CR, Kelleher AD. HIV vaccines: progress to date. *Drugs* 2011; 71: 387-414.

Neil SJD, McKnight A, Gustafsson K, Weiss, RA. HIV-1 incorporates ABO histo-blood group antigens that sensitize virions to complement-mediated inactivation. *Blood* 2005; 105: 4693-99.

Ni L, Ye F, Cheng ML, Feng Y, Deng YQ, Zhao H, et al. Detection of SARS-CoV-2-specific humoral and cellular immunity in COVID-19 convalescent individuals. *Immunity* 2020; 52: 971-77.

Ogawa H, Galili U. Profiling terminal N-acetyllactosamines of glycans on mammalian cells by an immuno-enzymatic assay. *Glycoconj J* 2006; 23: 663-74.

Parker W, Lin SS, Yu PB, Sood A, Nakamura YC, Song A, et al. Naturally occurring anti-α-galactosyl antibodies: Relationship to xenoreactive anti-α-galactosyl antibodies. *Glycobiology* 1999; 9: 865-73.

Pantaleo G, Koup RA. Correlates of immune protection in HIV-1 infection: what we know, what we don't know, what we should know. *Nat Med* 2004; 10: 806-10.

Pedro M, Folegatti PM, Katie J, Ewer KJ, Parvinder K, Aley P, et al. Safety and immunogenicity of the ChAdOx1 nCoV-19 vaccine against SARS-CoV-2: a preliminary report of a phase 1/2, single-blind, randomised controlled trial. *The Lancet* 2020; 396: 467-78.

Phelps CJ, Koike C, Vaught TD, Boone J, Wells KD, Chen SH, et al. Production of α1,3-galactosyltransferase-deficient pigs. *Science* 2003; 299: 411-14.

Pipperger L, Koske I, Wild N, Müllauer B, Krenn D, Stoiber H, et al. Xenoantigen-dependent complement-mediated neutralization of LCMV glycoprotein pseudotyped VSV in human serum. *J Virol* 2019; 93: e00567-19.

Pollack K, Zlotoff BJ, Borish LC, Commins SP, Platts-Mills TAE, Wilson JM. α-Gal Syndrome vs Chronic Urticaria. *JAMA Dermatol* 2019; 155: 115-16.

Portillo S, Zepeda BG, Iniguez E, Olivas JJ, Karimi NH, Moreira OC, et al. A prophylactic α-Gal-based glycovaccine effectively protects against murine acute Chagas disease. *NPJ Vaccines* 2019; 4: 13.

Posekany KJ, Pittman HK, Bradfield JF, Haisch CE, Verbanac KM. Induction of cytolytic anti-Gal antibodies in α-1,3-galactosyltransferase gene knockout mice by oral inoculation with *Escherichia coli* O86:B7 bacteria. *Infect Immun* 2002; 70: 6215-22.

Preece AF, Strahan KM, Devitt J, Yamamoto F, Gustafsson K. Expression of ABO or related antigenic carbohydrates on viral envelopes leads to neutralization in the presence of serum containing specific natural antibodies and complement. *Blood* 2002; 99: 2477-82.

Qiu JT, Song R, Dettenhofer M, Tian C, August T, Felber BK, et al., Evaluation of novel human immunodeficiency virus type 1 Gag DNA vaccines for protein expression in mammalian cells and induction of immune responses. *J Virol* 1999; 73: 9145-52.

Qiu Y, Xu MB, Yun MM, Wang YZ, Zhang RM, Meng XK, et al. Hepatocellular carcinoma-specific immunotherapy with synthesized α1,3-galactosyl epitope-pulsed dendritic cells and cytokine-induced killer cells. *World J Gastroenterol* 2011; 17: 5260-66.

Qiu Y, Yun MM, Xu MB, Wang YZ, Yun S. Pancreatic carcinoma-specific immunotherapy using synthesized α-galactosyl epitope-activated immune responders: findings from a pilot study. *Int J Clin Oncol* 2013; 18: 657-65.

Qiu Y, Yun MM, Dong X, Xu M, Zhao R, Han X, et al. Combination of cytokine-induced killer and dendritic cells pulsed with antigenic α-1,3-galactosyl epitope-enhanced lymphoma cell membrane for effective B-cell lymphoma immunotherapy. *Cytotherapy* 2016; 18: 91–8.

Regnault A, Lankar D, Lacabanne V, Rodriguez A, Théry C, Rescigno M, et al. Fcγ receptor-mediated induction of dendritic cell maturation and major histocompatibility complex class I-restricted antigen presentation after immune complex internalization. *J Exp Med* 1999; 189: 371-80.

Rossi GR, Mautino MR, Unfer RC, Seregina TM, Vahanian N, Link CJ. Effective treatment of preexisting melanoma with whole cell vaccines expressing α(1,3)-galactosyl epitopes. *Cancer Res* 2005; 65: 10555-61.

Rother RP, Fodor WL, Springhorn JP, Birks CW, Setter E, Sandrin MS, et al. A novel mechanism of retrovirus inactivation in human serum mediated by anti-α-galactosyl natural antibody. *J Exp Med* 1995; 182: 1345-55.

Rötzschke O, Falk K, Stevanović S, Jung G, Walden P, Rammensee HG, Exact prediction of a natural T cell epitope. *Eur J Immunol* 1991; 21: 2891-94.

Sandrin MS, Vaughan HA, Dabkowski PL, McKenzie IF. Anti-pig IgM antibodies in human serum react predominantly with Gal(α1-3)Gal epitopes. *Proc Natl Acad Sci USA* 1993; 90: 11391-95.

Shastri N, Gonzalez F. Endogenous generation and presentation of the ovalbumin peptide/Kb complex to T cells. *J Immunol* 1993; 150: 2724-36.

Schuurhuis DH, Ioan-Facsinay A, Nagelkerken B, van Schip JJ, Sedlik C, Melief CJ. Antigen-antibody immune complexes empower dendritic cells to efficiently prime specific CD8+ CTL responses in vivo. *J Immunol* 2002; 168: 2240-46.

Smith DF, Larsen RD, Mattox S, Lowe JB, Cummings RD. Transfer and expression of a murine UDP-Galβ-D-Gal-α1,3-galactosyltransferase gene in transfected Chinese hamster ovary cells. Competition reactions between the α1,3-galactosyltransferase and the endogenous α2,3-sialyltransferase. *J Biol Chem* 1990; 265: 6225-34.

Springer GF. Blood-group and Forssman antigenic determinants shared between microbes and mammalian cells. *Prog Allergy* 1971; 15: 9-77.

Stäger S, Alexander J, Kirby AC, Botto M, Rooijen NV, Smith DF, et al. Natural antibodies and complement are endogenous adjuvants for vaccine-induced CD8+ T-cell responses. *Nat Med* 2003; 9: 1287-92.

Stoner RD, Terres G. Enhanced antitoxin responses in irradiated mice elicited by complexes of tetanus toxoid and specific antibody. *J Immunol* 1963; 91: 761-70.

Stowell SR, Arthur CM, McBride R, Berger O, Razi N, Heimburg-Molinaro J, et al. Microbial glycan microarrays define key features of host-microbial interactions. *Nat Chem Biol* 2014; 10: 470-76.

Szymczakiewicz-Multanowska A, Groth N, Bugarini R, Lattanzi M, Casula D, Hilbert A, et al. Safety and immunogenicity of a novel influenza subunit vaccine produced in mammalian cell culture. *J Infect Dis* 2009; 200: 841-48.

Takeuchi Y, Porter CD, Strahan KM, Preece AF, Gustafsson K, Cosset FL, et al. Sensitization of cells and retroviruses to human serum by (α1-3) galactosyltransferase. *Nature* 1996; 379: 85-88.

Takeuchi Y, Liong SH, Bieniasz PD, Jäger U, Porter CD, Friedman T, et al. Sensitization of rhabdo-, lenti-, and spumaviruses to human serum by galactosyl(α1-3)galactosylation. *J Virol* 1997; 71: 6174-78.

Tanemura M, Maruyama S, Galili U. Differential expression of α-Gal epitopes (Galα1-3Galβ1-4GlcNAc-R) on pig and mouse organs. *Transplantation* 2000; 69: 187-90.

Tanemura M, Yin D, Chong AS, Galili U. Differential immune responses to α-gal epitopes on xenografts and allografts: implications for accommodation in xenotransplantation. *J Clin Invest* 2000; 105: 301-10.

Tearle RG, Tange MJ, Zannettino ZL, Katerelos M, Shinkel TA, Van Denderen BJ, et al. The α-1,3-galactosyltransferase knockout mouse. Implications for xenotransplantation. *Transplantation* 1996; 61: 13-19.

Teneberg S, Lönnroth I, Torres Lopez JF, Galili U, Olwegard Halvarsson M, Angstrom J, et al., Molecular mimicry in the recognition of glycosphingolipids by Galα3Galß4GlcNAcß-binding *Clostridium difficile* toxin A, human natural anti-α-galactosyl IgG and the monoclonal antibody Gal-13: characterization of a binding-active human glycosphingolipid, non-identical with the animal receptor. *Glycobiology* 1996; 6: 599-609.

Teranishi K, Manez R, Awwad M, Cooper DK. Anti-Gal α1-3Gal IgM and IgG antibody levels in sera of humans and Old World non-human primates. *Xenotransplantation* 2002; 9: 148-54.

Thall AD, Malý P, Lowe JB. Oocyte Galα1,3Gal epitopes implicated in sperm adhesion to the zona pellucida glycoprotein ZP3 are not required for fertilization in the mouse. *J Biol Chem* 1995; 270: 21437-40.

Towbin H, Rosenfelder G, Wieslander J, Avila JL, Rojas M, Szarfman A, et al. Circulating antibodies to mouse laminin in Chagas disease, American cutaneous leishmaniasis, and normal individuals recognize terminal galactosyl(α1-3)-galactose epitopes. *J Exp Med* 1987; 166: 419-32.

van Nunen S. Tick-induced allergies: mammalian meat allergy, tick anaphylaxis and their significance. *Asia Pac Allergy* 2015; 5: 3-16.

Vigerust DJ, Shepherd VL. Virus glycosylation: role in virulence and immune interactions. *Trends Microbiol* 2007; 15: 211-18.

Villinger F, Mayne AE, Bostik P, Mori K, Jensen PE, Ahmed R. Evidence for antibody-mediated enhancement of simian immunodeficiency virus (SIV) Gag antigen processing and cross presentation in SIV-infected rhesus macaques. *J Virol* 2003; 77: 10-24.

Walls AC, Tortorici MA, Frenz B, Snijder J, Li W, Rey FA, et al. Glycan shield and epitope masking of a coronavirus spike protein observed by cryo-electron microscopy. *Nat Struct Mol Biol* 2016; 23: 899-905.

Wan Y, Shang J, Graham R, Baric RS, Li F. Receptor recognition by the novel Coronavirus from Wuhan: an analysis based on decade-long structural studies of SARS Coronavirus. *J Virol* 2020; 94: e00127-20.

Wang L, Anaraki F, Henion TR, Galili U. Variations in activity of the human natural anti-Gal antibody in young and elderly populations. *J Gerontol Med Sci* 1995; 50A: M227–M233.

Wang M, Furnary AP, Li HF, Grunkemeier GL. Bioprosthetic aortic valve durability: A meta-regression of published studies. *Ann Thorac Surg* 2017; 104: 1080-87.

Wang S, Arthos J, Lawrence JM, Van Ryk D, Mboudjeka I, Shen S, et al. Enhanced immunogenicity of gp120 protein when combined with recombinant DNA priming to generate antibodies that neutralize the JR-FL primary isolate of human immunodeficiency virus type 1. *J Virol* 2005; 79: 7933-37.

Watanabe Y, Allen JD, Wrapp D, McLellan JS, Crispin M. Site-specific glycan analysis of the SARS-CoV-2 spike. *Science* 2020; 369: 330-33.

Webster RG. Immunity to influenza in the elderly. *Vaccine* 2000; 18: 1686-89.

Wei X, Decker JM, Wang S, Hui H, Kappes JC, Wu X, et al. Antibody neutralization and escape by HIV-1. *Nature* 2003; 422: 307-12.

Wei CJ, Boyington JC, Dai K, Houser KV, Pearce MB, Kong WP, et al. Cross-neutralization of 1918 and 2009 influenza viruses: Role of glycans in viral evolution and vaccine design. *Sci Transl Med* 2010; 2: 24ra21.

Welsh RM, O'Donnell CL, Reed DJ, Rother RP. Evaluation of the Galα1-3Gal epitope as a host modification factor eliciting natural humoral immunity to enveloped viruses. *J Virol* 1998; 72: 4650-56.

Whalen GF, Sullivan M, Piperdi B, Wasseff W, Galili U. Cancer immunotherapy by intratumoral injection of α-gal glycolipids. *Anticancer Res* 2012; 32: 3861-68.

Wiener AS, Origin of naturally occurring hemagglutinins and hemolysins; a review. *J Immunol* 1951; 66: 287-95.

Wigglesworth KM, Racki WJ, Mishra R, Szomolanyi-Tsuda E, Greiner DL, Galili U. Rapid recruitment and activation of macrophages by anti-Gal/α-Gal liposome interaction accelerates wound healing. *J Immunol* 2011; 186: 4422-32.

Wildt S, Gerngross TU. The humanization of N-glycosylation pathways in yeast. *Nat Rev Microbiol* 2005; 3: 119-28.

Wilson JM, Schuyler AJ, Schroeder N, Platts-Mills TA. Galactose-α-1,3-Galactose: Atypical food allergen or model IgE hypersensitivity? *Curr Allergy Asthma Rep*. 2017; 17: 8.

Wood C, Kabat EA, Murphy LA, Goldstein IJ. Immunochemical studies of the combining sites of the two isolectins, A4 and B4, isolated from *Bandeiraea simplicifolia*. *Arch Biochem Biophys* 1979; 198: 1-11.

Wrapp D, Wang N, Corbett KS, Goldsmith JA, Hsieh CL, Abiona O, et al. Cryo-EM Structure of the 2019-nCoV Spike in the prefusion conformation. *Science* 2020; 367: 1260-63.

Xiao C, Ling S, Qiu M, et al. Human post-infection serological response to the spike and nucleocapsid proteins of SARS-CoV-2 (published online ahead of print, 2020 Aug 25). *Influenza Other Respir Viruses*. 2020;10.1111/irv.12798. doi:10.1111/irv.12798.

Xie Y, Wang Z, Liao H, Marley G, Wu D, Tang W. Epidemiologic, clinical, and laboratory findings of the COVID-19 in the current pandemic: systematic review and meta-analysis. *BMC Infect Dis*. 2020; 20: 640.

Yan LM, Lau SPN, Poh CM, Chan VSF, Chan MCW, Peiris M, et al. Heterosubtypic protection induced by a live attenuated influenza virus vaccine expressing Galactose-α-1,3-Galactose epitopes in infected cells. *mBio* 2020; 11: e00027-20.

Yang TJ, Chang YC, Ko TP, Draczkowski P, Chien YC, Chang YC, et al. Cryo-EM analysis of a feline coronavirus spike protein reveals a unique structure and camouflaging glycans. *Proc Natl Acad Sci USA* 2020; 117: 1438-46.

Yilmaz B, Portugal S, Tran TM, Gozzelino R, Ramos S, Gomes J, et al. Gut microbiota elicits a protective immune response against malaria transmission. *Cell* 2014; 159: 1277-89.

Zinkernagel RM, Ehl S, Aichele P, Oehen S, Kündig T, Hengartner H. Antigen localization regulates immune responses in a dose- and time-dependent fashion: a geographical view of immune reactivity. *Immunol Rev* 1997; 156: 199-209.

Zhou P, Yang XL, Wang XG, Hu B, Zhang L, Zhang W, et al. A pneumonia outbreak associated with a new coronavirus of probable bat origin. *Nature* 2020; 579: 270-73.

In: Epidemics
Editor: Edward Paige
ISBN: 978-1-53618-976-6

Chapter 2

THE MYOPIA EPIDEMIC - A WORLDWIDE VISUAL CONCERN

Angie Wen, MD, David MacPherson, MD and Neesurg Mehta, MD
Department of Ophthalmology,
New York Eye and Ear Infirmary of Mount Sinai, New York, NY, US

ABSTRACT

Myopia is the most common ocular disorder worldwide. It is the leading cause of visual impairment in children, and the incidence is increasing rapidly. In 2010, an estimated 1.9 billion people (27% of the world's population) had myopia, 70 million of whom (2.8%) had high myopia, commonly defined as refractive error ≥ -6D. These numbers are projected to rise to 52% and 10%, respectively, by 2050. Vision impairment related to myopia has significant effects on a patient's quality of life, including physical, emotional, and social functioning. Pathologic myopia (prevalence 0.9%–3.1%), which confers an increased risk of cataract development, retinal detachment, glaucoma, and even blindness, is particularly devastating.

Major economic impact has resulted from the increasing prevalence of myopia. Experts have estimated the loss in world productivity caused by uncorrected myopia in 2004 to have been 268.8 billion international dollars and the cost of addressing this problem to be US $28 billion over 5 years.

Myopia is a particular public health concern in many East Asian countries, where the condition affects 80% to 90% of high school graduates. Of these individuals, 10% to 20% have sight threatening pathologic myopia. There appears to be not only environmental but also genetic factors that play a part in development and progression of myopia.

Initial research has shown that outdoor activity, sun light exposure, and low dose atropine all seem to help slow down the rate of myopia. It is theorized that visual input to the peripheral retina regulates adjacent scleral growth, and the relative peripheral hyperopic defocus in myopic eyes that remains despite wearing corrective myopic spectacles may be associated with elongation of the globe. Some have proposed using contact lenses that emphasize peripheral myopic defocus—and thus minimize hyperopic defocus—to help decrease progression of myopia. Similarly, there have been promising developments in technologies of lens spectacles to help slow down the rate of myopia. Perhaps the most exciting advancements have been in establishing efficacious dosing and drug delivery of low dose atropine to the pediatric population. The concern for this global epidemic of myopia has spurred intense research efforts, and there are a number of promising avenues for prevention and treatment.

INTRODUCTION

Epidemiology

The global myopia epidemic and its attendant visual consequences have been well established. There is a race to ameliorate that rise as incidence across the globe continues to increase at an alarming rate. Myopia is the most common disorder of the eye as well as the leading cause of visual impairment in children [1, 2]. Patients with myopia experience difficulty with focus on distance objects without appropriate corrective eyewear, which can interfere with daily activities such as learning in school or driving safely.

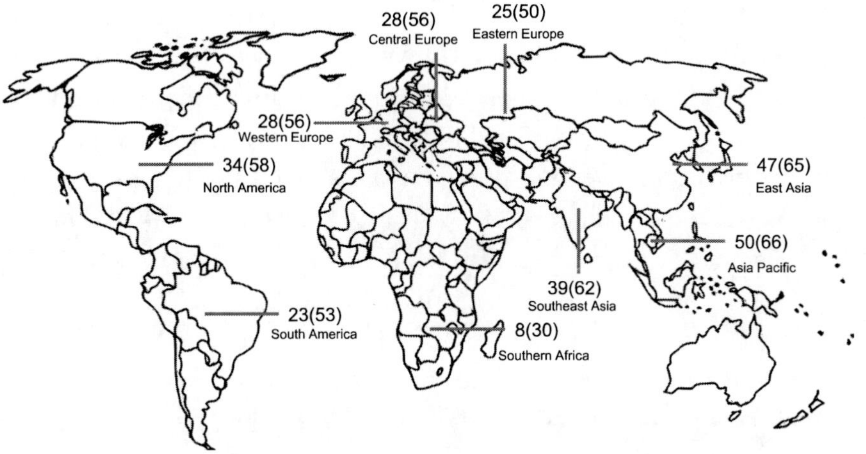

Figure. The Prevalence of Myopia Current % (Projected % in 2050).

The World Health Organization (WHO) defines myopia as spherical equivalent objective refractive error of ≤ –0.50 diopter in either eye, high myopia as ≥ –5.00 D in either eye, and myopic macular degeneration as refractive error ≥ –5.00 D with specific retinal changes, or refractive error ≥ –10.00 D with or without retinal changes [3].

According to data compiled from 145 studies including 2.1 million subjects, an estimated 22.9% of the world population had myopia and 2.7% had high myopia in the year 2000, with the largest cohort between 10-39 years old [1]. In addition, by the year 2050 it is projected that a staggering 49.8% of the world population will be myopic, with 9.8% of them high myopes [1] (see Figure).

The myopia epidemic is of particular concern in certain East Asian countries. For instance, in China and Taiwan, the disorder is estimated to affect 80-90% of high school graduates, 10-20% of whom have vision threatening pathologic myopia [2, 4]. According to Lam et al. the prevalence of myopia and high myopia in children age 6 was 18.3% and 0.7% respectively, and for those at age 12 was 61.5% and 3.8% [4].

In North America, the prevalence of myopia among high income families was estimated to be 28.3% in 2000 and projected to be 58.4% in 2050 [1]. In the United States, analysis of the IRIS (Intelligent Research in Sight) Data registry and the NHANES (National Health and Nutrition

Examination Survey) data revealed diopter-adjusted prevalence of high myopia in 2014 to be 3.92% in 2014 with prevalence of pathologic myopia of 0.33% [5]. A cross sectional study of pediatric patients in Southern California by Theophanous shed light on the breakdown of myopia among age groups and race/ethnic background. Myopia was found to be more common in older children (59% in ages 17-19 versus 14.8% in those between 5 and 7 years of age) [6]. Household income was found to play a role as median households with income of $25,000 -$40,000 had lower rates of myopia compared to households with incomes less than 25,000 [6]. In addition, patients of Asian/Pacific Islander descent had an increased rate of myopia compared to their Caucasian and African American counterparts [6].

Wen et al. looked at the prevalence of myopia in a multi-ethnic pediatric eye disease study and found that non-Hispanic white children had the lowest overall prevalence of myopia compared to the other four racial/ethnic groups studied, whereas children of Asian descent had the highest prevalence [7]. However, no difference was found between gender in the children included in the study.

Sequelae of Myopia

There are significant visual complications associated with myopia, in particular pathologic myopia, which has an estimated prevalence of 0.9%-3.1% [3, 8]. Among the many sequelae are cataract, retinal damage including choroidal neovascularization and retinal detachment, glaucoma, and blindness. The WHO notes that the most common cause of vision impairment is undercorrected myopia likely from lack of access to providers and resources for corrective eyewear [3]. While corrective eyewear can remedy simple myopia and cataracts can be removed with surgery, the peripheral vision loss that occurs with glaucomatous optic nerve damage and the central vision loss that occurs with Myopic Macular Degeneration [MMD] of the retina is unfortunately permanent. Glaucoma involves progressive damage to the optic nerve fiber layer and loss of peripheral vision that can eventually affect central vision if left untreated. MMD can be seen clinically as either patchy or diffuse chorioretinal atrophy. In advanced cases, abnormal blood vessel development, known as choroidal neovascularization (CNV), can develop in the fovea of the retina, which is responsible for central vision [3]. These abnormal blood vessels leak blood and proteins into the surrounding retina and can cause vision loss and distortion. The prevalence of CNV in individuals with MMD is estimated to be 5.2% to 11.3%, and can be bilateral in 30% of patients. Macular holes, which can be particularly damaging to central vision, can occur in 6% to 8% of these cases [8, 9].

As previously mentioned, the burden of disease is increased in patients of Asian descent. An estimated 1% of Caucasian compared to 1-3% of Asians counterparts have pathologic myopia [3, 8]. Furthermore, pathologic myopia in Asians leads to more visual impairment and blindness compared to Caucasians [3, 8].

Financial Burden of Myopia

The myopia epidemic also has significant global economic consequences. Poor vision resulting from myopia leads to loss of work force and inefficiencies in the work and home environment. According to Fricke, uncorrected refractive error contributes to a loss of $202 billion of the global gross domestic product [10]. In addition, it is estimated that there was a loss in world productivity of 268.8 billion international dollars in 2004, and it cost 28 billion US dollars to address the issue [11]. The astounding burden disproportionally affects people from low-income families [12]. Additionally, a study by Ma et al. in China suggests that providing access to refractive correction in low socioeconomic areas would improve educational outcomes in children [13].

In Singapore the direct cost attributed to remedy myopia per child per year is estimated to be $148 US dollars [14]. Zheng et al. looked at 125 myopic patients and found the mean cost per person per year was $709 US dollars and a lifetime per capita cost of $17,020 for those with an 80-year lifespan. A breakdown of the cost estimate includes such services as glasses, contact lenses, refractive surgery, and overall ophthalmologic services [15].

PATHOGENESIS

Onset/Progression

The onset of myopia seems to increase significantly after the age of 6. This increase has previously been linked in studies to the beginning of school and attendant increase in near work and hours spent studying [16, 17]. The prevalence rate of myopia in subjects less than 6 years of age tends to be less than 5% even in areas of high burden such as East Asia [18-21]. However, the incidence in even this very young population is increasing as well. Fa et al. found an estimated increase in myopia of 6.3% from 2.3% over 10 years among Hong Kong preschoolers [22].

In Chinese populations the annual incidence of myopia between the ages of 7-15 years has been relatively constant with up to 80% of certain subpopulations suffering from myopia [23]. Studies show comparable patterns in other East Asian countries, with increased incidence at even younger ages suggested in Singapore, Taiwan, and Hong Kong [24-26]. Western countries seem to fare better, with meta-analyses showing a much lower childhood incidence of myopia with a later age onset as well [27]. Rahi et al. reported that most cases of myopia identified in the United Kingdom were in children 16 years of age or older [28].

The meta-analysis performed by Rudnicka et al. reported that populations in South Asia, black populations in Africa, and Hispanics tended to have lower prevalence of myopia than Western white populations, whereas black populations outside of Africa, South-East Asians, Middle Eastern/North African populations, Native Hawaiians, and American Indians have a higher prevalence [27]. All these groups still have significantly lower incidence of myopia compared with East Asian populations [27].

Environment

The alarming rise of myopia has led investigators to work to uncover modifiable risk factors for myopia in order to engage in early prevention. Multiple risk factors contributing to the development of myopia have been postulated. Among those explored are time spent outdoors, near work, and a societal shift to dependence on phones, tablets, and computers.

At the current time, the predominant protective environmental factor seems to be time spent outdoors. A potential dose dependent relationship has been researched between the amount of time spent outdoors and the risk of myopia [29, 30]. In a systematic review Xiong et al. looked at the relationship between outdoor time with the incidence of myopia as well as progression in already myopic eyes. There was a protective effect against myopia *onset* with increased time spent outdoors. Unfortunately, there was no effect on slowing progression in patients *already* myopic [29]. The study elucidated the need for further investigation on the subject including optimal time outdoors and strategies for implementing this protective environmental factor. The authors acknowledged multiple limitations of the study including retrospective nature and high heterogeneity among the studies analyzed.

The hypothesized mechanism of protection of time spent outdoors include biochemical activity, a uniform dioptric space, relaxed accommodation and increased pupil constriction, as well as physical activity [30]. Light stimulated retinal release of dopamine and other neurotransmitters that inhibit increased axial length may serve as the biochemical mechanism for decreased myopia with outdoor activity [30, 31]. This has been supported to some degree in certain animal studies while other mechanisms explaining outdoor time protection have had less of an impact [30, 31]. Outdoor sports and other physical activity have been theorized to contribute to decreased incidence of myopia. Interestingly, a study by Rose et al. found that there was no association between participating in indoor sports and myopia [32]. Further studies attempting to separate the factors of increased light exposure and outdoor/indoor activity would be of great interest in guiding recommendations for children and physical education classes in school.

Near Work

Another environmental factor highly investigated in association with myopia is near work. The definition of and means of measurement of near work has been highly variable among different studies. This included level of education, duration of sustained study time, duration of leisure reading, books read per certain amount of time, font size, and screen use [33].

Near work as a cause of myopia is especially problematic given that over the last two decades, daily routine in many developed countries has shifted exponentially towards the reliance on digital formats for work, leisure, and activities of daily living. Much of this digital content is consumed on screens at arm's length, such as on smartphones and desktop or tablet computers. Communication has transitioned heavily to texting, emails, and video usage, all which require sustained near work activity. This dependence on screen time contributes to increased cumulative near work hours. Huang et al. found in a systematic review and meta-analysis of 12 cohort studies and 15 cross-sectional studies that increased time spent participating in near work activity was associated with higher odds of myopia, and that the odds of developing myopia increased by 2% for every additional diopter-hour of near work performed per week [34].

Even more worrisome is the fact that children are introduced to screen time via phones and tablets at a younger and younger age as forms of early education and entertainment. The Sydney Vascular and Eye Study (SAVES) was a 5 to 6 year follow up study of 2103 children that showed an increased odds of incidence of myopia by age 12 for those children with short periods of time outdoors and longer duration and frequency of near work [30]. A Study in Shanghai by You examined the relationship between various near work activities among 6-to-10-year-old children and myopia over a one year follow up [35]. In the study, the participants and their parents filled out a questionnaire together on nine different near work factors in addition to baseline eye exams which included measurements such as axial length and cycloplegic refraction at baseline and one year follow up. They reported on various factors that were associated with increased myopia as measured by both cycloplegic refraction and axial length biometry. These included use of an inappropriate distance with the eye while reading, writing, or engaging in TV screen time, poor lighting while reading or writing, and continuous near work greater than 30-40 minutes without an eye break [35].

The Covid19 pandemic and the attendant recommendations for social distancing have resulted in a shift to working from home for many adults, and remote learning for children, resulting in an exponential increase in screen time for both groups. There is great concern that a semi-permanent switch to digital classrooms can have a devastating acceleration in the rise of myopia in young children. Currently, the WHO and the American Academy of Pediatrics recommend no screen time at all for children younger than 2 years of age, and less than 1 hour a day for children 2 to 5 years old [36]. More studies are required in the future to study the effects of digital near work on children and adolescents, especially those of handheld devices.

Genetics

Genetic factors and hereditability have also been explored in the development of myopia. More than 150 gene loci associated with myopia have been identified in genome-wide association studies [37]. A study by Chen reported nine gene loci that were associated with axial length RSPO1, C3orf26, LAMA2, GJD2, ZNRF3, CD55, MIP, ALPPL2, and ZC3H11B [38]. The researchers organized the mentioned loci into two groups. The first group includes loci involved in the Wnt signaling pathway related to the regulation of axial length (RSPO1 and ZNRF3). The other group includes 5 loci that were found to be associated with common refractive error variation *LAMA2, GJD2, CD55, ALPPL2*, and *ZC3H11B.*

A meta-analysis by Sanfilippo reported that hereditability for refractive error was 0.71 [39]. Other heritability estimates from studies have ranged from 0.11 to 0.98, the higher estimate coming from a study of Finnish female twins [40]. Although many gene loci have been identified, genetic risk scores estimate they only explain 0.6% of the variance in refractive error at age 7 and only 2.3% at age 15 [43].

Family history of myopia has also been investigated. Zhang et al. summarized in a meta-analysis an association between the number of myopic parents and incident myopia [43]. The odds ratios calculated in this analysis ranged from 1.44 to 2.96 for having a myopic child depending on the number of myopic parents [43]. Another study of Chinese students found that there were 26-fold higher odds for prevalent myopia in students with close reading distances and two parents with myopia [44]. However, family history as a risk factor has further indications, particularly in light of increased myopic prevalence. Xiang comments that the odds of a child becoming myopic with two myopic parents is different than the odds of a myopic child having parents that are both myopic because there are likely more children than parents with myopia [45]. Thus, the sensitivity of parental myopia in predicting childhood myopia remains weak [46].

TREATMENT

Contact Lenses

It is theorized that input to the peripheral retina regulates adjacent scleral growth, and in turn the peripheral hyperopic defocus associated with globe elongation and thus myopia [47, 48]. Consequently, there is interest in using contact lenses that emphasize peripheral myopic defocus to help counteract hyperopic defocus and to decrease myopic progression. Early studies have been promising, with Lam of Hong Kong finding a 25% slower progression of myopia with specialty bifocal defocus-incorporated soft contact lenses compared with single-vision soft contact lenses. This treatment effect had a positive correlation with length of time the defocus-incorporated soft contact lenses were used [49].

A review by Bullimore looked at multiple treatment methods researched in the prevention of myopia, including soft contact lenses that alter central distance zone and provide increased peripheral retina positive power [50]. Variables manipulated among studies included lens design, amount of power provided by the lens periphery, spherical area of positive power, multiple concentric treatment zones, and spherical aberration. They concluded that while single vision soft contact lenses were not recommended in myopic children, multifocal and orthokeratology lenses could potentially become the standard of care for preventing myopic progression in children and adolescents.

A study by Walline looked at progression of axial length and myopia among eight-to-eleven-year old children fitted with distance center soft multifocal contact lenses over a two year period [51]. It was found that myopia and axial length progression were decreased in participants by 50% and 29% respectively. Another study found similar progression reduction in dual-focus soft contact lenses among participants eleven to fourteen years of age. It was reported that in 70% of the children enrolled in the study, myopic progression was reduced by 30% in those assigned to dual focus lenses [52].

A study among Chinese children ranging from ages seven to fourteen by Sankaridurg found that reducing relative peripheral hyperopia with contact lenses can slow progression of axial length and myopia as well [53]. They reported that the spherical equivalent at 12 months was 34% less (-0.57D in contact lenses versus -0.86 D glasses) and that axial length was 33% less in those in the contact lens group.

Orthokeratology

Orthokeratology involves the placement of a hard gas permeable contact lens overnight to temporarily alter the cornea curvature to improve visual acuity throughout the day. Previous studies have shown temporary improvement of visual acuity, though there is expected regression of the majority of the effects during the day when the lens is not worn. Current research focus has turned to the potential of orthokeratology in reducing myopic progression. A randomized trial of 78 participants by Cho and Cheung over a two year period found a reduced increase in axial length by 43% in those assigned to orthokeratology compared to those wearing single-vision glasses over time [54]. In addition, it was reported that younger participants had faster rates of axial elongation suggesting earlier initiation of treatment. A study by Li estimated the two year reduction in axial length progression to be around 0.28mm [55].

A study by Santodomingo-Rubido looked at the increase in axial length over a seven year period in a group of subjects wearing orthokeratology lenses compared to controls. Rate of change in axial length was reported to be 33% less in those patients using orthokeratology lenses [56]. Another prospective study over five years found a statistically significant difference in axial length between orthokeratology versus control groups [57]. Axial length during the 5 years was 0.99 ± 0.47 for the orthokeratology group and 1.41 ± 0.68 mm for the control group. It must be noted that there are considerable safety concerns associated with orthokeratology including but not limited to the potential for blinding microbial keratitis associated with overnight contact lens wear, and thus the use of orthokeratology at all is still considered controversial in many medical ophthalmologists [58, 59].

MiSight

MiSight dual-focused optical design soft contact lenses by Cooper Vision (USA) are the first contact lenses approved by the FDA for reducing myopia in November 2019. The study performed in 2018 showed a significant slowing of the progression of myopia and axial length over a four year time period including in children starting use at later ages [60].

A three year multicenter randomized clinical trial of MiSight lenses was conducted by Chamberlain comparing the dual-focus MiSight lens with a single-vision contact lens of the same material and general geometry. Overall, it was reported that MiSight was effective in slowing the progression of spherical equivalence and axial length in the participants ages eight to twelve years old. Spherical equivalent refraction was found to be 59% less in the MiSight group than the control group (−0.51 ± 0.64 vs. –1.24 ± 0.61 D, $P < .001$) [61]. In addition, mean change in axial length was also found to be 52% less in the MiSight group (0.30 ± 0.27 vs. 0.62 ± 0.30 mm, $P < .001$). A two year study performed in Spain by Ruiz-Pomeda looked at MiSight compared to single vision contact lenses, and reported similar findings that the MiSight group had a slower progression of myopia and decreased axial elongation compared to the control single-vision contact lens wearers [62].

Spectacles

Glasses have also been an area of interest in efforts to slow the myopia epidemic, though many studies have not found clinically significant reductions. The COMET (Correction of Myopia Evaluation Trial) was a landmark study that compared progression of myopia in subjects using progressive addition lenses (PALs) and single vision lenses. PALs are lenses that have a blended bifocal design with the top segment of the lens used for distance focus, and progressively positive lens power towards the bottom of the lens with corresponding shorter and shorter focal points. It was found that myopia progression was slowed in subjects in the PALs group compared to the group with single vision lenses. A 5 year follow up of the COMET study found only a small statistically significant difference between the groups that was present only during the first year [63]. Edwards reported a similar disappointing finding in progressive addition lenses versus single vision lenses. After two years they found that there was no difference in axial length or myopic progression between the two groups [64].

Bifocal glasses have also been evaluated in reducing accommodative lag and hyperopic focus to reduce myopia. In a three year randomized control trial by Cheng et al. subjects were assigned to one of three groups, single vision glasses, +1.50 D bifocals, or +1.50 bifocals with 3 D base down prism in the near segment. It was reported that both bifocals and prismatic bifocals significantly slowed myopia progression compared to single-vision lenses during the study time period [65]. Average spherical equivalents reported over the three years were -2.06 D for single-vision lens, -1.25 D for bifocal, and -1.01 D for the bifocal plus prism group.

Other research in spectacles is ongoing, many through innovative biotech companies. SightGlass Vision (USA) is currently working on developing novel spectacles aimed at slowing myopia progression in children. The CYPRESS (Control of Myopia Using Peripheral Diffusion Lenses: Efficacy and Safety Study) trial is an ongoing multicenter, double-masked, randomized controlled clinical trial that is looking to measure myopia progression over the course of 36 months using novel lens designs [66].

The Defocus Incorporated Multiple Segments (DIMS) spectacle lens (Hoya Vision, Japan) is a specialized lens that features a central optical zone that corrects refractive error and includes multiple microlenses around the central zone and extending to the midperiphery that produce constant myopic defocus. A 2 year double masked randomized controlled trial by Lam et al. looked at 160 Chinese children aged 8 to 13 years who had between -1.00 and -5.00 D of myopia and 1.50 D or less of astigmatism. The results showed that children wearing DIMS lenses myopia progressed 52% slower and had 62% less axial length elongation compared to the single vision glasses group over the two year period [67]. Furthermore, seventeen of the 79 children (21.5%) in the DIMS group and six of the 81 children (7%) in the single vision group had no myopia progression during the 2-year study.

Atropine

Medical therapy has been at the forefront of myopia prevention, with the antimuscarinic agent atropine being an especially promising medication under investigation. Atropine is a cycloplegic agent that dilates the pupil and restricts accommodation. Accommodation is the process by which the eye changes from distance focus to near focus, and involves changes in the natural eye lens shape and contraction and relaxation of the ciliary muscle. Although the exact mechanism of action of slowing myopic progression is unclear, some postulate an anti-muscarinic impact on receptors in scleral fibroblasts that slow axial length elongation [68, 69].

A study by Shih from 2001 was important in showing that atropine had a greater therapeutic effect for myopic progression than glasses. In this randomized clinical trial, the results from 188 myopic children assigned to three groups 0.5% atropine with multi-focal glasses, multifocal glasses, and single vision spectacles over an 18 month period were provided. Main conclusions from the study were that myopia progression was significantly correlated with increased axial length, those assigned to the 0.5% atropine and multifocal lens group had a significant reduction in myopia progression, and that multi-focal lenses failed to show difference in effect compared to control [70].

The ATOM1 (Atropine for Treatment of Childhood Myopia study) by Chu et al. looked at 346 children aged 6 to 12 over two years who were randomly assigned to 1% atropine drops or control vehicle drops. There was a reduction in progression of myopia of -0.92D and reduction in axial length elongation of 0.40mm in groups treated with atropine 1% compared with control [68]. ATOM2, a follow-up study, further investigated the effective dose-dependence of atropine in preventing myopia progression [69]. 400 children were randomly assigned in a 2:2:1 ratio to 0.5%, 0.1%, and 0.01% atropine drops. Mean myopia progression at 2 years was found to be -0.30 ± 0.60, -0.38 ± 0.60, and -0.49 ± 0.63 D in the atropine 0.5%, 0.1%, and 0.01% groups, respectively, and the mean increase in axial length was 0.27 ± 0.25, 0.28 ± 0.28, and 0.41 ± 0.32 mm respectively [69]. Differences in myopia progression and axial length between groups however were not found to be clinically significant. Furthermore, it was found that there was a rapid rebound increase in myopia when atropine was stopped for 12 months after the 24 months of study treatment. The group receiving atropine 0.01%, had the least rebound effect and had minimal side effects compared to the 0.1% and 0.5% groups, suggesting extended efficacy of a low-dose of atropine [69] (see Table).

The more recent LAMP (The Low-Concentration Atropine for Myopia Progression) study took a closer look at even lower doses of atropine, investigating safety and efficacy of atropine at 0.05%, 0.025%, and 0.01% concentrations compared to placebo over a 1-year period [71]. Subjects were randomly assigned in a 1:1:1:1 ratio to receive 0.05%, 0.025%, 0.01%, or placebo nightly. All atropine concentrations were found to slow myopic progression, with the 0.05% being the most effective in reducing progression of both spherical equivalent and axial length elongation [71].

Study	Year/Authors	Key Findings
An intervention trial on efficacy of atropine and multi-focal glasses in controlling myopic progression	2001/ Shih et al.	0.5% atropine with multi-focal lenses can slow down the progression rate of myopia Multi-focal lenses alone showed no difference in effect compared to single vision lenses (control)
Atropine for Treatment of Childhood Myopia study (ATOM1)	2006/ Chua et al.	Reduction in progression of myopia of -0.92D and reduction in axial length elongation of 0.40mm in groups treated with atropine 1% compared with control
Atropine for the treatment of childhood myopia: safety and efficacy of 0.5%, 0.1%, and 0.01% doses (Atropine for the Treatment of Myopia 2) (ATOM2)	2012/ Chia et al.	Differences in myopia progression and axial length change between groups were small and clinically insignificant Atropine 0.01% has minimal side effects compared with atropine at 0.1% and 0.5
Five-Year Clinical Trial on Atropine for the Treatment of Myopia 2: Myopia Control with Atropine 0.01% Eyedrop	2016/ Chia et al.	Medications were stopped for 12 months after the initial 24 months of study treatment, and the group receiving atropine 0.01%, had the least rebound effect and had minimal side effects compared to the 0.1% and 0.5% groups
The Low-Concentration Atropine for Myopia Progression (LAMP) Study: Phase 2 Report	2020/ Yam et al.	0.05%, 0.025%, and 0.01% atropine eye drops were all well tolerated and reduced myopia progression along a concentration-dependent response 0.05% atropine was most effective in controlling spherical equivalent progression and axial elongation

A recent randomized clinical trial conducted by Wei et al. in published in October 2020 sought to determine the safety and efficacy of atropine 0.01%. 220 Chinese children aged 6 to 12 were randomly assigned in a 1:1 ration to atropine 0.01% or placebo groups. Results after 1 year showed a relative reduction of myopic progression of 34.2% and 22.0% in axial elongation in the group receiving 0.01% atropine [72].

Since the ideal window for treatment for myopia prevention appears to be in the pediatric age group, there is also a push to research novel methods of medication administration to make it more tolerable for children, who often find eyedrop application uncomfortable. The Optejet dispenser by EyeNovia (USA) uses piezo-print technology to allow children to self-administer 8 μL of atropine in order to minimize dose-related side effects [73]. Their ongoing CHAPARONE study, a US-based phase 3 multicenter, randomized, double-masked study, seeks to investigate the safety and efficacy of the Optejet dispenser, enrolling more than 400 children.

Pirenzepine

Another drug being investigated for myopia prevention is pirenzepine, a relatively selective antimuscarinic M1- receptor antagonist. Atropine is a nonselective antimuscarinic agent. A study by Siatkowski randomized children aged 8 to 12 years in a 2:1 ratio to receive 2% pirenzepine ophthalmic gel or placebo twice daily. At 1 year, the mean increase in myopia om the pirenzepine group compared to control was 0.26 D and 0.53 D respectively. At 2 years, the mean increase in myopia was 0.58 D and 0.99 for the pirenzepine group and the placebo group respectively [74].

Conclusion

The myopia epidemic is sweeping the globe at an alarming rate with potential visual consequences that impact productivity and individual quality of life. With such profound visual, social, and economic consequences, the importance of mitigating progression has never been greater. Further research needs to be conducted on modifiable environmental risk factors, genomics, and medical therapy. Higher near work demands in our increasingly digital world threatens to accelerate the rise in prevalence of myopia. Dual zone contact lenses and other specialty contact lenses and spectacles seem to be promising treatments. Atropine in particular is a major focus of pharmacological treatment. In addition, continued innovation in providing therapy and reaching those communities most at risk must be implemented.

References

[1] Fricke TR, Jong M, Naidoo KS, et al. Global prevalence of visual impairment associated with myopic macular degeneration and temporal trends from 2000 through 2050: systematic review, meta-analysis and modelling. *Br J Ophthalmol*. 2018;102(7):855-862.

[2] Ma Y, Qu X, Zhu X, et al. Age-specific prevalence of visual impairment and refractive error in children aged 3-10 years in Shanghai, China. *Invest Ophthalmol Vis Sci.* 2016;57(14):6188-6196.

[3] The impact of myopia and high myopia. Report of the Joint World Health Organization–Brien Holden Vision Institute Global Scientific Meeting on Myopia. University of New South Wales, Sydney, Australia, March 16-18, 2015. Geneva: *World Health Organization*; 2017. License: CC BY-NC-SA 3.0 IGO. https://www.who.int/blindness/causes/MyopiaReportforWeb.pdf. Accessed June 25, 2019.

[4] Lam CS, Lam CH, Cheng SC, Chan LY. Prevalence of myopia among Hong Kong Chinese schoolchildren: changes over two decades. *Ophthalmic Physiol Opt* 2012;32:17-24.

[5] Willis JR, Vitale S, Morse L, et al. The Prevalence of Myopic Choroidal Neovascularization in the United States: Analysis of the IRIS(®) Data Registry and NHANES. *Ophthalmology*. 2016;123(8):1771-1782. doi:10.1016/j.ophtha.2016.04.021.

[6] Theophanous, C., Modjtahedi, B. S., Batech, M., Marlin, D. S., Luong, T. Q., & Fong, D. S. (2018). Myopia prevalence and risk factors in children. *Clinical ophthalmology* (Auckland, N. Z.), 12, 1581–1587. https://doi.org/10.2147/OPTH.S164641.

[7] Wen, G., Tarczy-Hornoch, K., McKean-Cowdin, R., Cotter, S. A., Borchert, M., Lin, J., Kim, J., Varma, R., & Multi-Ethnic Pediatric Eye Disease Study Group (2013). Prevalence of myopia, hyperopia, and astigmatism in non-Hispanic white and Asian children: multi-ethnic

pediatric eye disease study. *Ophthalmology*, 120(10), 2109–2116. https://doi.org/10.1016/j.ophtha.2013.06.039.

[8] Wong TY, Ferreira A, Hughes R, Carter G, Mitchell P. Epidemiology and disease burden of pathologic myopia and myopic choroidal neovascularization: an evidence-based systematic review. *Am J Ophthalmol*. 2014;157(1):9-25.e12.

[9] Ohno-Matsui K, Yoshida T, Futagami S, Yasuzumi K, Shimada N, Kojima A. Patchy atrophy and lacquer cracks predispose to the development of choroidal neovascularisation in pathological myopia. *Br J Ophthalmol*. 2003;87:570–3.

[10] Fricke TR, Holden BA, Wilson DA, Schlenther G, Naidoo KS, Resnikoff S, Frick KD *Bull World Health Organ*. 2012 Oct 1; 90(10):728-38.

[11] Smith TS, Frick KD, Holden BA, Fricke TR, Naidoo KS. Potential lost productivity resulting from the global burden of uncorrected refractive error. *Bull World Health Organ*. 2009;87(6):431-437.

[12] Global magnitude of visual impairment caused by uncorrected refractive errors in 2004. Resnikoff S, Pascolini D, Mariotti SP, *Pokharel GP Bull World Health Organ*. 2008 Jan; 86(1):63-70.

[13] Ma X, Zhou Z, Yi H, Pang X, Shi Y, Chen Q et al. Effect of providing free glasses on children's educational outcomes in China: cluster randomized controlled trial. *BMJ*. 2014;349:g5740.

[14] Lim MC, Gazzard G, Sim EL, Tong L, Saw SM. Direct costs of myopia in Singapore. *Eye*. 2009;23:1086–9.

[15] Zheng YF, Pan CW, Chay J, Wong TY, Finkelstein E, Saw SM. The economic cost of myopia in adults aged over 40 years in Singapore. *Invest Ophthalmol Vis Sci*. 2013;54(12):7532-7537. Published 2013 Nov 13. doi:10.1167/iovs.13-12795.

[16] Ma Y, Qu X, Zhu X, et al. Age-specific prevalence of visual impairment and refractive error in children aged 3-10 years in Shanghai, China. *Invest Ophthalmol Vis Sci*. 2016; 57: 6188–6196.

[17] Morgan IG, Rose KA. Myopia and international educational performance. *Ophthalmic Physiol Opt*. 2013; 33: 329–338.

[18] James S. Wolffsohn, Daniel Ian Flitcroft, Kate L. Gifford, Monica Jong, Lyndon Jones, Caroline C. W. Klaver, Nicola S. Logan, Kovin Naidoo, Serge Resnikoff, Padmaja Sankaridurg, Earl L. Smith, David Troilo, Christine F. Wildsoet; IMI – Myopia Control Reports Overview and Introduction. *Invest. Ophthalmol. Vis. Sci.* 2019;60(3):M1-M19. doi: https://doi.org/10.1167/iovs.18-25980.

[19] Fan DS, Cheung EY, Lai RY, Kwok AK, Lam DS. Myopia progression among preschool Chinese children in Hong Kong. *Ann Acad Med Singapore*. 2004; 33: 39–43.

[20] Dirani M, Zhou B, Hornbeak D, et al. Prevalence and causes of decreased visual acuity in Singaporean Chinese preschoolers. *Br J Ophthalmol.* 2010; 94: 1561–1565.

[21] Lan W, Zhao F, Lin L, et al. Refractive errors in 3-6 year-old Chinese children: a very low prevalence of myopia? *PLoS One.* 2013; 8: e78003.

[22] Fan DS, Lai C, Lau HH, Cheung EY, Lam DS. Change in vision disorders among Hong Kong preschoolers in 10 years. *Clin Exp Ophthalmol.* 2011; 39: 398–403.

[23] Wu JF, Bi HS, Wang SM, et al. Refractive error, visual acuity and causes of vision loss in children in Shandong, China: The Shandong Children Eye Study. *PLoS One*. 2013; 8: e82763.

[24] Jung SK, Lee JH, Kakizaki H, Jee D. Prevalence of myopia and its association with body stature and educational level in 19-year-old male conscripts in Seoul, South Korea. *Invest Ophthalmol Vis Sci.* 2012; 53: 5579–5583.

[25] Koh V, Yang A, Saw SM, et al. Differences in prevalence of refractive errors in young Asian males in Singapore between 1996-1997 and 2009-2010. *Ophthalmic Epidemiol*. 2014; 21: 247–255.

[26] Lam CS, Goldschmidt E, Edwards MH. Prevalence of myopia in local and international schools in Hong Kong. *Optom Vis Sci*. 2004; 81: 317–322.

[27] Rudnicka AR, Kapetanakis VV, Wathern AK, et al. Global variations and time trends in the prevalence of childhood myopia, a systematic

review and quantitative meta-analysis: implications for aetiology and early prevention. *Br J Ophthalmol.* 2016; 100: 882–890.

[28] Rahi JS, Cumberland PM, Peckham CS. Myopia over the lifecourse: prevalence and early life influences in the 1958 British birth cohort. *Ophthalmology*. 2011; 118: 797–804.

[29] Xiong S, Sankaridurg P, Naduvilath T, et al. Time spent in outdoor activities in relation to myopia prevention and control: a meta-analysis and systematic review. *Acta Ophthalmol*. 2017;95(6):551-566.

[30] French AN, Ashby RS, Morgan IG, Rose KA. Time outdoors and the prevention of myopia. *Exp Eye Res*. 2013;114:58-68.

[31] Carr BJ, Stell WK. The science behind myopia. In: Kolb H, Nelson R, Fernandez E, Jones B, eds. *Webvision: The Organization of the Retina and Visual System*. University of Utah Health Sciences Center. https://webvision.med.utah.edu/book/part-xvii-refractive-errors/the-science-behind-myopia-by-brittany-j-carr-and-william-k-stell. Accessed June 25, 2019.

[32] Rose, KA, IG Morgan, J. Ip, A. Kifley, S. Huynh, W. Smith, P. Mitchell Outdoor activity reduces the prevalence of myopia in children. *Ophthalmology*, 115 (2008), pp. 1279-1285.

[33] Wolffsohn, JS, Flitcroft, DI, Gifford, KL, Jong, M, Jones, L, Klaver, C, Logan, N. S, Naidoo, K, Resnikoff, S, Sankaridurg, P, Smith, E. L, 3rd, Troilo, D., & Wildsoet, C. F. (2019). IMI - Myopia Control Reports Overview and Introduction. *Investigative ophthalmology & visual science*, 60(3), M1–M19.

[34] Huang HM, Chang DS, Wu PC. The association between near work activities and myopia in children-a systematic review and meta-analysis. *PLoS One*. 2015; 10: e0140419.

[35] You X, Wang L, Tan H, He X, Qu X, Shi H, Zhu J, Zou H. Near Work Related Behaviors Associated with Myopic Shifts among Primary School Students in the Jiading District of Shanghai: A School-Based One-Year Cohort Study. *PLoS One*. 2016 May 3;11(5):e0154671. doi: 10.1371/journal.pone.0154671. PMID: 27139017; PMCID: PMC4854402.

[36] Cimberle, M. Increased digital screen time during COVID-19 may accelerate myopia epidemic. *Ocular Surgery News*. helio.com/news/ophthalmology/20201014/increased-digital-screen-time-during-covid19-may-acclerate-myopia-epidemic. Accessed Oct 20, 2020.

[37] Williams KM, Hysi P, Hammond CJ. Twin studies, genome-wide association studies and myopia genetics. *Ann Eye Sci*. 2017; 2: 69.

[38] Cheng, CY, Schache, M, Ikram, MK, Young, TL, Guggenheim, JA, Vitart, V, MacGregor, S, Verhoeven, VJ, Barathi, VA, Liao, J, Hysi, PG, Bailey-Wilson, JE, St Pourcain, B, Kemp, JP, McMahon, G, Timpson, NJ, Evans, DM, Montgomery, GM, Mishra, A, Wang, Y. X, … Baird, PN. (2013). Nine loci for ocular axial length identified through genome-wide association studies, including shared loci with refractive error. *American journal of human genetics*, 93(2), 264–277.

[39] Sanfilippo PG, Hewitt AW, Hammond CJ, Mackey DA. The heritability of ocular traits. *Surv Ophthalmol*. 2010; 55: 561–583.

[40] Angi MR, Clementi M, Sardei C, Piattelli E, Bisantis C. Heritability of myopic refractive errors in identical and fraternal twins. *Graefes Arch Clin Exp Ophthalmol*. 1993; 231: 580–585.

[41] Teikari JM, Kaprio J, Koskenvuo MK, Vannas A. Heritability estimate for refractive errors—a population-based sample of adult twins. *Genet Epidemiol*. 1988; 5: 171–181.

[42] Fan Q, Guo X, Tideman JW, et al. Childhood gene-environment interactions and age-dependent effects of genetic variants associated with refractive error and myopia: *The CREAM Consortium. Sci Rep*. 2016; 6: 25853.

[43] Zhang X, Qu X, Zhou X. Association between parental myopia and the risk of myopia in a child. *Exp Ther Med*. 2015; 9: 2420–2428.

[44] Si JK, Tang K, Bi HS, Guo DD, Guo JG, Wang XR. Orthokeratology for myopia control: a meta-analysis. *Optom Vis Sci*. 2015; 92: 252–257.

[45] Xiang F, He M, Morgan IG. Annual changes in refractive errors and ocular components before and after the onset of myopia in Chinese children. *Ophthalmology*. 2012; 119: 1478–1484.

[46] Wenbo L, Congxia B, Hui L. Genetic and environmental-genetic interaction rules for the myopia based on a family exposed to risk from a myopic environment. *Gene*. 2017; 626: 305–308.

[47] Smith EL III, Hung LF, Arumugam B. Visual regulation of refractive development: insights from animal studies. *Eye* (Lond). 2014;28(2): 180-188.

[48] Yeo A, Paillé D, Drobe B, Koh P. Myopia and effective management solutions. *Points de Vue.* www.pointsdevue.com/ article/myopia-and-effective-management-solutions. Accessed July 8, 2019.

[49] Lam CS, Tang WC, Tse DY, Tang YY, To CH. Defocus incorporated soft contact (disc) lens slows myopia progression in Hong Kong Chinese schoolchildren: a 2-year randomised clinical trial. *Br J Ophthalmol*. 2014;98(1):40-45.

[50] Bullimore MA, Richdale K. Myopia Control 2020: Where are we and where are we heading? *Ophthalmic & Physiological Optics: the Journal of the British College of Ophthalmic Opticians* (Optometrists). 2020 May;40(3):254-270. DOI: 10.1111/opo.12686.

[51] 51 Walline JJ, Greiner KL, McVey ME & Jones-Jordan LA. Multifocal contact lens myopia control. *Optom Vis Sci* 2013; 90: 1207–1214.

[52] 52. Anstice NS & Phillips JR. Effect of dual-focus soft contact lens wear on axial myopia progression in children. *Ophthalmology* 2011; 118: 1152–1161.

[53] 53. Sankaridurg P, Holden B, Smith E 3rd et al. Decrease in rate of myopia progression with a contact lens designed to reduce relative peripheral hyperopia: one-year results. *Invest Ophthalmol Vis Sci* 2011; 52: 9362–9367.

[54] 54. Cho P & Cheung SW. Retardation of myopia in Orthokeratology (ROMIO) study: a 2-year randomized clinical trialized clinical trial. *Invest Ophthalmol Vis Sci* 2012; 53: 7077–7085.

[55] 55. Li SM, Kang MT, Wu SS et al. Efficacy, safety and acceptability of orthokeratology on slowing axial elongation in myopic children by meta-analysis. *Curr Eye Res* 2016; 41: 600–608.

[56] 56. Santodomingo-Rubido J, Villa-Collar C, Gilmartin B et al. Long-term Efficacy of Orthokeratology Contact Lens Wear in Controlling the Progression of Childhood Myopia. *Curr Eye Res* 2017; 42: 713–720.

[57] 57. Hiraoka T, Kakita T, Okamoto F et al. Long-term effect of overnight orthokeratology on axial length elongation in childhood myopia: a 5-year follow-up study. *Invest Ophthalmol Vis Sci* 2012; 53: 3913–3919.

[58] 58. VanderVeen DK, Kraker RT, Pineles SL, et al. Use of orthokeratology for the prevention of myopic progression in children: a report by the American Academy of Ophthalmology. *Ophthalmology*. 2019;126(4):623-636.

[59] 59. Kam KW, Yung W, Li GKH, Chen LJ, Young AL. Infectious keratitis and orthokeratology lens use: a systematic review. *Infection*. 2017;45(6):727-735.

[60] *CooperVision releases four-year data on landmark MiSight 1 Day Contact Lens Study; pioneering approach slows myopia progression in children* [press release]. Singapore: CooperVision; September 18, 2018. https://coopervision.com/our-company/news-center/press-release/coopervision-releases-four-year-data-landmark-misight-1-day. Accessed June 25, 2019.

[61] Chamberlain P, Peixoto-de-Matos SC, Logan NS et al. A 3-year randomized clinical trial of MiSight lenses for myopia control. *Optom Vis Sci* 2019; 96: 556–567.

[62] Ruiz-Pomeda A, Perez-Sanchez B, Valls I et al. MiSight Assessment Study Spain (MASS). A 2-year randomized clinical trial. *Graefes Arch Clin Exp Ophthalmol* 2018; 256: 1011–1021.

[63] Gwiazda J, Hyman L, Hussein M et al. A randomized clinical trial of progressive addition lenses versus single vision lenses on the progression of myopia in children. *Invest Ophthalmol Vis Sci* 2003; 44: 1492–1500.

[64] Edwards MH, Li RW, Lam CS et al. The Hong Kong progressive lens myopia control study: study design and main findings. *Invest Ophthalmol Vis Sci* 2002; 43: 2852–2858.

[65] Cheng D, Woo GC, Drobe B & Schmid KL. Effect of bifocal and prismatic bifocal spectacles on myopia progression in children: three-year results of a randomized clinical trial. *JAMA Ophthalmol* 2014; 132: 258–264.

[66] *SightGlass Vision multicenter trial to study novel eyeglasses to control nearsightedness for FDA approval* [news release]. Palo Alto, CA: PRNewswire; January 10, 2019. https://prnmedia.prnewswire.com/news-releases/sightglass-vision-multicenter-trial-to-study-novel-eyeglasses-to-control-nearsightedness-for-fda-approval-300776509.html. Accessed June 25, 2019.

[67] Lam CSY, Tang WC, Tse DY, et al. Defocus incorporated multiple segments (DIMS) spectacle lenses slow myopia progression: a 2-year randomised clinical trial [published online ahead of print May 29, 2019]. *Br J Ophthalmol*. doi: 10.1136/bjophthalmol-2018-313739.

[68] Chua WH, Balakrishnan V, Chan YH, et al. Atropine for the treatment of childhood myopia. *Ophthalmology*. 2006;113(12):2285-2291.

[69] Chia A, Chua WH, Cheung YB, et al. Atropine for the treatment of childhood myopia: safety and efficacy of 0.5%, 0.1%, and 0.01% doses (Atropine for the Treatment of Myopia 2). *Ophthalmology*. 2012;119(2):347-354.

[70] Shih YF, Hsiao CK, Chen CJ et al. An intervention trial on efficacy of atropine and multi-focal glasses in controlling myopic progression. *Acta Ophthalmol Scand* 2001; 79: 233–236.

[71] Yam JC, Jiang Y, Tang SM, et al. Low-Concentration Atropine for Myopia Progression (LAMP) Study: a randomized, double-blinded, placebo-controlled trial of 0.05%, 0.025%, and 0.01% atropine eye drops in myopia control. *Ophthalmology*. 2019;126(1):113-124.

[72] Wei S, Li S, An W, et al. Safety and Efficacy of Low-Dose Atropine Eyedrops for the Treatment of Myopia Progression in Chinese Children: A Randomized Clinical Trial. *JAMA Ophthalmol*. Published online October 01, 2020. doi:10.1001/jamaophthalmol. 2020.3820.

[73] *Eyenovia enrolls first patient in phase III CHAPERONE Study for progressive myopia* [news release]. New York: Globe Newswire; June 4, 2019. www.globenewswire.com/news-release/2019/06/04/1863

931/0/en/Eyenovia-Enrolls-First-Patient-in-Phase-III-CHAPERONE-Study-for-Progressive-Myopia.html. Accessed June 25, 2019.

[74] Siatkowski RM, Cotter SA, Crockett RS et al. Two-year multicenter, randomized, double-masked, placebo-controlled, parallel safety and efficacy study of 2% pirenzepine ophthalmic gel in children with myopia. *J AAPOS* 2008; 12: 332–339.

In: Epidemics
Editor: Edward Paige
ISBN: 978-1-53618-976-6

Chapter 3

DETECTING AND PREVENTING WHEAT STRIPE RUST EPIDEMICS IN ARGENTINA

***Marcelo Carmona*[1], *Francisco Sautua*[1] *and Oscar Pérez-Hérnandez*[2]**
[1]Facultad de Agronomía, Cátedra de Fitopatología, Universidad de Buenos Aires, Ciudad Autónoma de Buenos Aires, Argentina
[2]School of Agricultural Sciences, Northwest Missouri State University, Maryville, MO, US

ABSTRACT

Wheat stripe rust (SR), caused by the fungus *Puccinia striiformis* f. sp. *tritici* (*Pst*), is one of the most aggressive crop diseases worldwide that threatens global food security. In Argentina, the disease caused the worst epidemics in 2017 affecting about three million hectares. The occurrence of the epidemics was anomalous, as for 87 years there had not been disease outbreaks of this magnitude. We were able to relate the epidemics to the incursion of new exotic strains of *Pst* into the Argentine wheat-growing regions, where the majority of wheat varieties are susceptible to the disease. In addition, we estimated the impact and chemical control of the disease in the region. Average wheat yield losses were estimated at 3,700 kg ha^{-1} (53%) in field trials conducted in the epidemic area with a maximum of up to 4,700 kg ha^{-1} (70%) in the seven most susceptible varieties. This scenario represents a challenge for plant breeders, since the vast majority of wheat varieties are susceptible to the new *Pst* races. Fungicides showed to be highly effective in reducing SR intensity and yield losses, thus they have become the only tool for managing SR when planting SR-susceptible wheat varieties. In this work, we analyze the importance of detection and prevention of SR epidemics in Argentina under the described scenario and within the context of an integrated management of the disease.

Keywords: yellow rust, *Puccinia striiformis* f. sp. *tritici*, epidemiology, fungicides

INTRODUCTION

Importance of Wheat Stripe Rust

Wheat stripe rust (SR), caused by *Puccinia striiformis* Westend. f. sp. *tritici* Erikss (*Pst*), was first described by Gadd and Bjerkander in Europe in 1777 (Eriksson and Henning, 1896) and is widespread in all the wheat-growing regions of the world. Currently, SR is one of the most important and destructive diseases of wheat worldwide. The disease can cause up to 70% yield losses in highly susceptible wheat varieties (Chen and Kang, 2017a). Global yield losses were estimated at more than 5 million tons and annual economic losses at USD 1 billion (Beddow et al., 2015). Historically, wheat stem rust, caused by *Puccinia graminis* Pers. f. sp. *tritici* Eriks. & E. Henn. (*Pgt*), was considered the rust that caused the greatest losses in wheat crops (Beddow et al., 2015). However, in recent years, SR became the disease causing the greatest losses due to the recent epidemics registered around the world (Chen and Kang, 2017a). The SR causal agent, *Pst*, is an obligate biotrophic parasite that has a high variability and adaptability, continuously mutating into new races or pathotypes. This phenomenon is the main cause of the different wheat varieties genetic resistance breakdown by *Pst*. It is estimated that 88% of the world's wheat production is currently vulnerable to the pathogen (Beddow et al., 2015; Schwessinger, 2016).

Because of all of the aforementioned characteristics, SR may be considered as the main phytosanitary challenge of wheat cultivation worldwide at present (Hovmøller et al., 2010, Chen et al., 2014, Beddow et al., 2015, Schwessinger, 2016).

The species of rust fungus *P. striiformis* is divided into several formae speciales (special forms) based on host specialization, i.e., varieties within this species (based on host specificity and/or morphological characteristics). It can infect different cereals such as wheat (*P. striiformis* f. sp. *tritici*), barley (*P. striiformis* f. sp. *hordei*), rye (*P. striiformis* f. sp. *secalis*), and different grasses such as *Agropyron* spp. (*P. striiformis* f. sp. *agropyri*) and *Elymus* spp. (*P. striiformis* f. sp. *elymi*) (Chen and Kang, 2017a; Huang et al., 2019). *Pst* is classified as a typical heteroecious, macrocyclic rust since the alternate hosts (*Berberis* spp. and *Mahonia* spp.) were recently identified (Jin et al., 2010; Wang and Chen, 2013). This discovery allows to ponder the impact of potential sexual recombination in generating new and more aggressive strains of the pathogen (Zhao et al., 2016; Mehmood et al., 2020a,b). For the case of Argentina, however, this aspect is unknown and there is no evidence to support that the sexual cycle of *Pst* actually occurs in nature in the Southern Cone of South America. Future research will be key in elucidating this unknown. The urediniospores (asexual spores of the pathogen) can be dispersed by wind over long distances and are responsible for severe epidemics that develop on wheat crops (Hovmøller et al., 2002). Therefore, it is believed that survival and initial inocula of wheat rusts occur on self-sown (voluntary) wheat plants in Argentina and neighbour countries at latitudes where frost does not occur during the off-season.

The SR epidemics that occurred in Argentina during the 2017/2018 growing season, coupled with the resulting yield losses, situate SR as one of the most economically important diseases of wheat in the country. This stems from the fact that wheat is the main cereal crop in the country, with a cultivated area of 6.7 million hectares and a total production of 18.5 million tons, per year (MINAGRI, 2018). This chapter describes how SR became the most important disease in Argentina upon the incursion of new (exotic) pathogenic *Pst* races into the country. The chapter also addresses how detection and prevention of epidemics play a crucial role in SR integrated management.

Detection and Diagnosis of SR

In general, the geographic location and prevalence of rusts that attack cereals largely depend on the average temperature, the susceptibility of the wheat genotypes that are planted and the races of the pathogen present in each particular growing season. In Argentina, the three rusts that infect wheat are present. The most important is SR (Figures 1 to 6). The second in importance is leaf rust, caused by *Puccinia triticina* Eriks., which is common and endemic to South America (Figures 7 and 8) (Lindquist, 1982; Carmona et al., 2000, German et al., 2007).

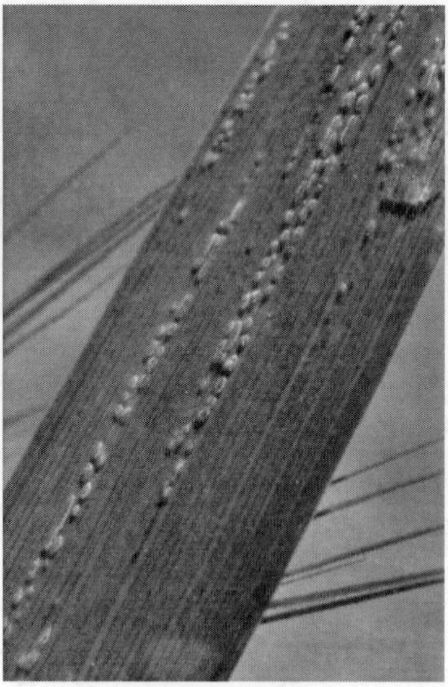

Figure 1. Signs (uredosoric pustules) of stripe rust (SR), caused by *Puccinia striiformis* f. sp. *triticina* (Pst). Author: Di Nubila S., Carmona M.

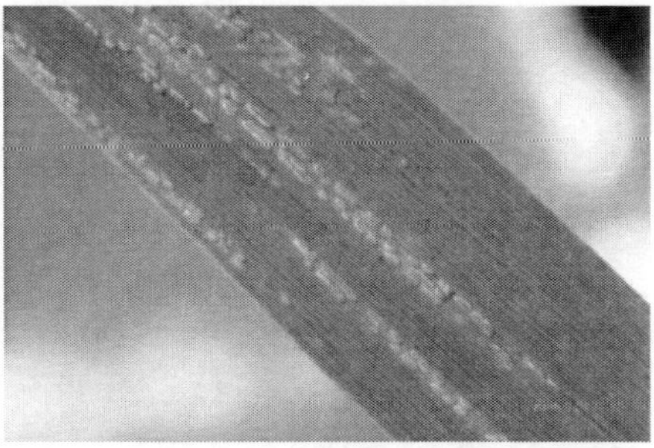

Figure 2. Signs and symptoms (chlorosis) of SR in a highly susceptible wheat variety in Argentina. Author: Di Nubila S., Carmona M.

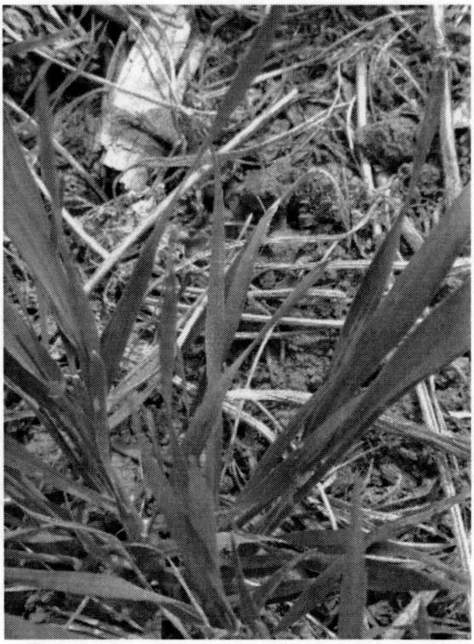

Figure 3. Pustules of SR in early vegetative stages of wheat in Argentina. Author: Vettorello L.

Finally, not less important is the stem rust, caused by *Pgt*, which can cause devastating epidemics in few days when infecting susceptible varieties (Figures 9 and 10) (Carmona et al., 2020). Leaf rust occurs more frequently than stem rust, but the prevalence and severity of the latter has increased in the last growing seasons in the Argentine Pampas region.

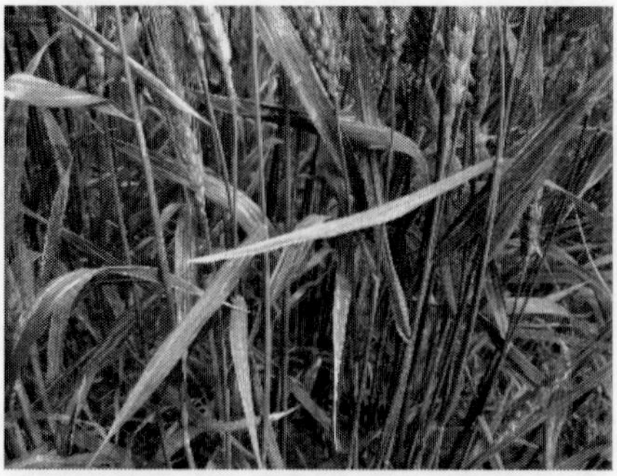

Figure 4. Pustules of SR are arranged in lines between leaf veins. Author: Carmona M.

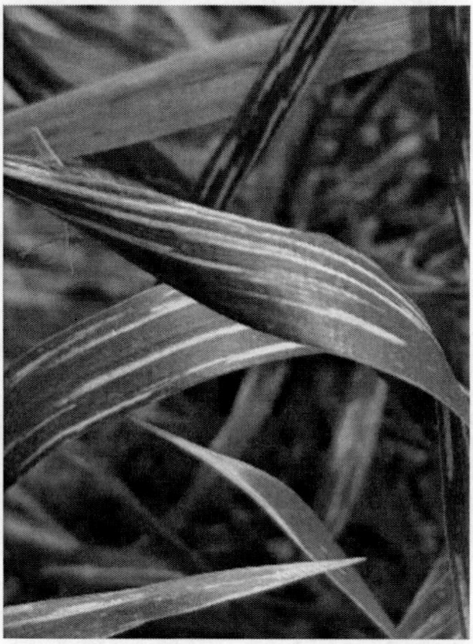

Figure 5. Necrotic stretch marks of SR after fungicide application in Argentina. Author: Carmona M.

Wheat rusts are easy to distinguish between each other and from other wheat diseases, particullary when the pustules are young. The differences between the three rusts are summarized in Table 1. SR pustules are yellow orange arranged in stripes on leaves (Figure 1). When the disease becomes severe in susceptible varieties, SR can develop on glumes, lemma, palea and awns. The characteristic yellow color can be more easily distinguished during the morning because most spores are produced overnight (Stubbs,

1985; Chen, 2005). Generally, pustules are arranged in lines between leaf veins (Figure 2).

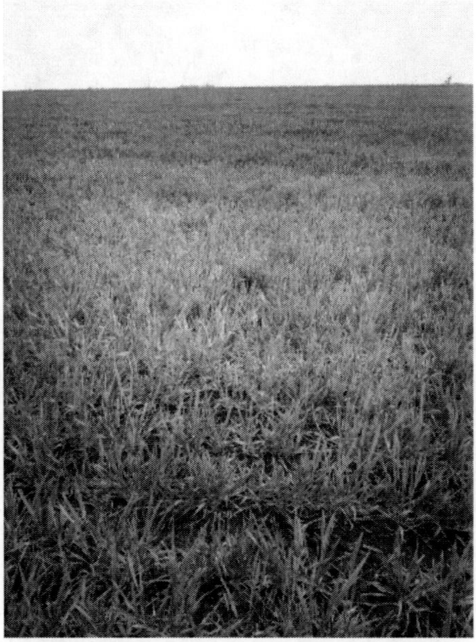

Figure 6. Hot spot of SR in the field in Argentina. Author: Vettorello L.

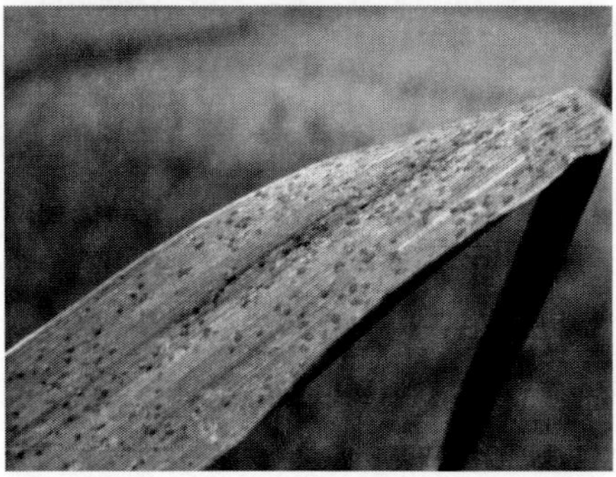

Figure 7. Leaf rust pustules caused by *Puccinia triticina* in Brasil. Author: Reis E.M.

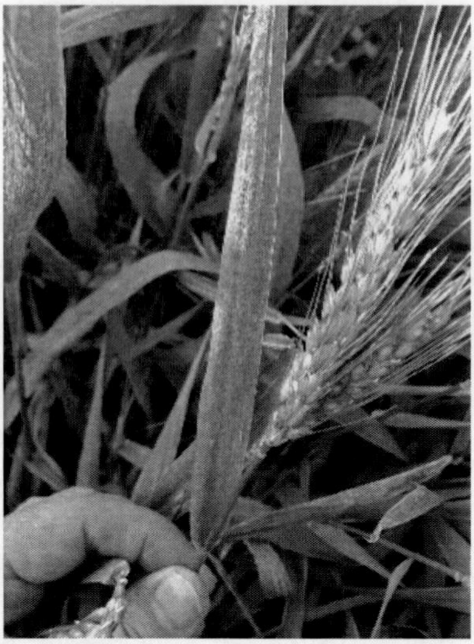

Figure 8. Leaf rust pustules caused by *Puccinia triticina* in a highly susceptible wheat variety in Argentina. Author: Vettorello L.

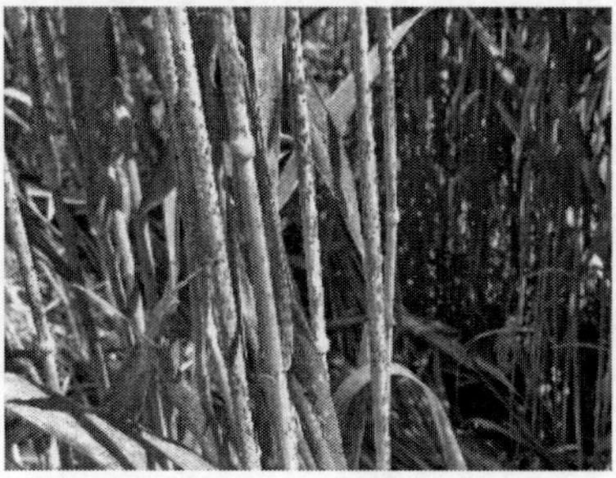

Figure 9. Stem rust pustules, caused by *Puccinia graminis* f. sp. *tritici*, in Argentina. Author: Carmona M.

However, sometimes uredinia do not appear in linear arrangement, especially in the seedling stage of some cultivars, and could cause the diagnosis to be difficult when trying to distinguish between SR from leaf rust (Figure 3). The same happens when the infection is very severe on the leaves of adult plants where the density of pustules does not allow to clearly distinguish the stripes (Figure 4) (Cheng, 2020). Dead stripes without pustules can often be observed on some leaves, especially after a late fungicide application or in varieties that show some type of resistance (Figure 5). Later, the teleutosoric pustules appear with black teleutospores that are also arranged in the form of stripes. These pustules tend to be more frequently arranged on the upper side of the leaves.

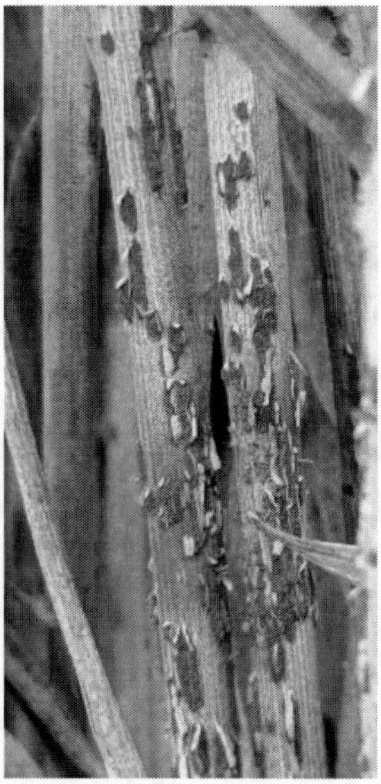

Figure 10. Stem rust pustules in a highly susceptible wheat variety in Argentina. Author: Carmona M.

The interaction between the host plant (wheat), the pathogenic organism (causative agents of rusts) and the environment is visibly expressed through signs (pustules) and symptoms (chlorosis). These vary from its absence (immune wheat variety) to its maximum manifestation (susceptible cultivars). Symptoms and signs, therefore, are used to quantify these diseases. The number of pustules per leaf or the percentage of covered leaf area expresses the severity of the disease, while the percentage of plants or leaves attacked represents the incidence. The intensity of the disease is a function of the incidence and severity. The more susceptible the cultivar, the more virulent the rust races will be and if the environmental conditions are optimal for the development of the disease, then the maximum values of severity and incidence will be reached (Reis and Carmona, 2000).

Table 1. Hosts and symptoms of leaf, stem and stripe rusts

Disease	Pathogen	Primary (uredinial/telial) hosts	Alternate (pycnial/aecial) hosts	Uredospores on primary host[6]	Teliospores on primary host[6]	Symptoms
Leaf rust	*Puccinia triticina* (*Pt*)	Common wheat (*Triticum aestivum* L.), durum wheat (*T. turgidum* L. var. *durum*), cultivated emmer wheat (*T. dicoccon*) and wild emmer wheat (*T. dicoccoides*), *Aegilops speltoides*, goatgrass (*Ae. cylindrica*), and triticale (X Triticosecale) [1]	*Thalictrum speciosissimum* (= *T. flavum glaucum*), *Isopyrum fumaroides* [1]	20-28 x 18-21 µm and have a diameter of 15 to 30 µm, subglobose and orange or reddish brown in color, with three to eight germinating pores distributed in their thick equinulate walls.	36-65 x 11-22 µm, bicellular, ellipsoidal, clavulate and pointed.	Typical leaf rust. Isolated or scattered uredinia on upper leaf surface.
Stem rust	*Puccinia graminis* f. sp. *tritici* (*Pgt*)	Common wheat (*Triticum aestivum* L.), durum wheat (*T. turgidum* L. var. *durum*), cultivated barleys (*Hordeum vulgare* L.), triticale (X Triticosecale) [2]	Barberry (*Berberis* spp.), Oregon grape (*Mahonia* spp.), and their hybrids (× *Mahoberberis*) [4]	17-25 x 18-22 µm, reddish orange, dehiscent and oblong oval.	39-57 X 15 X 18 µm, rounded and flattened at their apices, transversely septate into two cells, the lower one shortly pedicellate	Frequently on stem and spikes (glume and awns). Isolated uredinia on upper and lower leaf surfaces.

Table 1. (Continued)

Disease	Pathogen	Primary (uredinial/telial) hosts	Alternate (pycnial/aecial) hosts	Uredospores on primary host[6]	Teliospores on primary host[6]	Symptoms
Stripe rust	*Puccinia striiformis* f. sp. *tritici* (*Pst*)	Common wheat (*Triticum aestivum* L.), durum wheat (*T. turgidum* var. *durum* L.), cultivated emmer wheat (*T. dicoccum* Schrank), wild emmer wheat (*T. dicoccoides* Korn), triticale (X Triticosecale), cultivated barleys (*Hordeum vulgare* L.), rye (*Secale cereale* L.), naturalized and improved pasture grass species (*Elymus canadensis* L., *Leymus secalinus* Hochst, *Agropyron* spp. Garetn, *Hordeum* spp. L., *Phalaris* spp. L, *Bromus unioloides* Kunth) [3]	Barberry (*Berberis chinensis*, *B. koreana*, *B. holstii*, *B. vulgaris*, *B. shensiana*, *B. potaninii*, *B. dolichobotrys*, *B. heteropoda*, etc.) and Oregon grape (*Mahonia aquifolium*, *Mahonia* spp., etc.)[3,5]	23-35 x 20-31 µm and have a diameter of 20 to 30 µm, yellowish orange, with thick walls equinulated with 6 to 12 germinative pores.	35-63 x 12-20 µm, subepidermal, frequently on sheaths, clavulate, with rounded apex, similar to those of *P. triticina*	Systemic uredinia on leaves (stripes) and spikes (glumes and awns)

Source: modified from Roelfs et al., 1992.[1] Bolton et al., 2008.[2] *Pgt* was shown to infect 74 species in 34 genera in artificial inoculations of seedlings, but only 28 of those species belonging to eight genera were known to be natural hosts of the fungus (Leonard and Szabo, 2005).[3] Chen et al., 2014.[4] More than 90 species or varieties of *Berberis*, *Mahonia*, and their hybrids (× *Mahoberberis*) have been found to be susceptible to *P. graminis*; being *Berberis vulgaris* the most important species in North America and Europe (Roelfs, 1985).[5] At present, 33 species of *Berberis* and *Mahonia* have been reported to be susceptible to *Pst* (Zhao et al., 2016).[6] indquist, 1982; Bushnell and Roelfs, 1984; Carmona et al., 2000.

In the particular case of SR, unlike other wheat rusts, at the beginning of the epidemics it is common to observe the symptoms and signs of the disease distributed in groups of few plants in the field, developing the typical infected patches known as "foci" or hot-spots (Figure 6). They can be seen in the distance as islands of yellowish spots or patches, up to 10 meters in diameter, in the middle of a wheat field. The foci pattern in hot spots would appear to be due to a combination of spore biology and morphology, moisture in the atmosphere and to greater susceptibility of upper leaves (Farber et al., 2017). If there is a high relative humidity, as it is frequent in winters of Argentina, most of the urediniospores are grouped together and remain in the air in small groups: they are relatively heavy and quickly fall out of the air, so their propagation takes place mainly over very short distances, generating so-called "hot spots" or foci. These hot-spots or patches can often be mistaken for nutrient deficiencies, waterlogging, or soil defects. Therefore, it is essential that when scouting, disease scouting be directed specifically at those spots. Because of the SR latent period (the time it takes for a spore to penetrate and infect until new pustules with uredinisopores are produced), which usually takes between 10 to 14 days, it is very likely that after observing hot-spots, most plants in a whole field plot are infected. On the contrary, if there is not high relative humidity in the air, spores are dispersed in the air in an ungrouped manner and can travel considerably longer distances. This can give a uniform infection or generalized disease pattern development and not patches. SR spreads rapidly in the field and readily to other leaves and plants as infection of susceptible wheat varieties by *Pst* is highly effective. The proximity between wheat plants at normal planting densities (200-300 plants m^2) facilitates natural infection and consequently increases the epidemic rate of development.

The dispersal of urediniospores can be attributed to wind and rainsplash. Rains can favor the disease not because of its gravitational impact, but because they can guarantee humid hours to facilitate germination. However, excessive or intense rains could eliminate the spore stock in the air (Geagea et al., 1999). Urediniospores of SR can be spread by the wind from a few meters to more than 8000 km in the same growing season (Chen and Kang, 2017a; (Brown and Hovmøller, 2002). They have an adherent mucilaginous membrane and therefore can be dispersed mainly as groups of 2 to 10 spores (Rapilly et al., 1970). In contrast, spores of *Pgt* and *Pt* are mainly removed and dispersed as single spores (Geagea et al., 1997). According to Geagea et al. (1997), wind speed is very efficient at removing *Pst* urediniospores from diseased leaves at a speed of between 3 and 5 m s^{-1}. This dispersal ability causes fields to turn "yellow" in a few days, showing a large number of infected and sporulated wheat leaves. However, viable urediniospores are frequently dispersed within a certain region but may not be successful in initiating an epidemic. This is because wheat cultivars from that region may be resistant to the predominant genotype of the pathogen, environmental conditions after dissemination may be unfavorable or spores may arrive late with no time for the development of the epidemic.

Spore transport through human travel by aircraft can also contribute to the spread of the pathogen between countries. A clearly example was carried out by Wellings (2007) who demonstrated the introduction of Pst into Australia in 1979 from Europe, through contaminated passenger clothing.

Occurrence and Development Epidemics of SR in Argentina

According to available historical records, *Pst* was first reported in South America in the early 20th century, with an unknown origin (Rudorf and Job, 1934; Stubbs, 1985). Nevertheless, according to recent multilocus microsatellite genotyping studies, it is hypothesized that *Pst* migrated to South America from northwestern Europe in the early 1900s, probably through human intervention and not by wind (Ali et al., 2014). In Argentina, SR first appeared in 1929 attacking almost 80% of the total wheat grown area (Humphey and Crowell, 1930). The following year the disease caused severe epidemics causing losses estimated at 2 million tons, representing 30% of the total production of that year (Fernández Valiela, 1979; Lindquist, 1982). At that time, Humphey and Crowell (1930) suggested the possibility of SR being brought into the country from Europe in shipments containing wheat plant material with urediniospores.

According to these authors, the disease was registered in an area of about 10 million hectares. The Tres Arroyos area located southeast of the province of Buenos Aires was one of the most attacked wheat regions at that time. In that location, there were two periods of disease attack: at the beginning of flowering (Zadocks 6.1 stage), by initial infections on lower leaves, and a more severe attack at the milky grain stage (Zadocks 7.5 stage). The spread of the epidemic was favored by the susceptibility of the varieties planted at that time (examples are Klein Record and Klein San Martín). High grain losses caused by SR forced growers to replace the most susceptible (and most planted) wheat varieties to the least susceptible (Fernández Valiela, 1979). Since 1930, the disease had only been sporadic and especially confined to regions with cooler temperatures in the southern wheat growing area of Buenos Aires province (German et al., 2007). Thus, Argentina was historically considered marginally favorable for the epidemic development of SR due to its climate, except for the southern region of the Buenos Aires province with cooler average temperatures.

After almost 90 years of no epidemic occurrence, the agronomic scenario changed due to the introduction into the country of new races, virulent to the majority of Argentine wheat varieties. It was during the 2017/2018 and 2018/2019 growing seasons that SR was observed in regions with higher mean temperatures than those in south of the Buenos Aires province, where it had not been previously reported. The disease caused serious and widespread epidemics in many wheat growing regions of Argentina, especially in fields with high-water content soils and frequent dew formation. In total, more than 3 million hectares were affected including warmer areas of the Argentine Pampas for the first time. Unusual and early infections of SR were detected at several locations in the Entre Rios, Córdoba, Santa Fe, and Buenos Aires provinces. Typical "foci" or hot-spots were observed at the beginning of epidemics. The disease spread rapidly throughout most wheat-growing areas of the country and the SR was observed on almost all wheat cultivars (Carmona et al., 2019). During these two growing seasons, the Plant Pathology Department of the FAUBA coordinated a *Pst* survey in the Argentine Pampas region.

During the first year of sampling, the SR foliar severity ranged from 5% to 50% depending on the particular crop environment and wheat variety. The maximum was registered in Pergamino, Buenos Aires (33°54'59.15"S; 60°27'30.92"W), and the minimum in Landeta, Santa Fe (31°59'00"S; 62°01'36"W). In the second year of sampling, SR foliar severity ranged from <1% in Alejo Ledesma (33°40'51.36"S, 62°37'49.48"W), Ordoñez (32°55'05.36"S, 62°53'59.71"W) and Oro Verde (31°51'24", 60°38'22"), to 80% in Famaillá, Tucumán (27°03'14"S; 65°24'11"W). Likewise, samples of Triticale and Candeal wheat affected by SR were detected with a severity range of 1 to 5%.

Argentine *Pst* genetic lineages were analyzed by the Global Rust Reference Center (Aarhus University, Denmark). Annually, the GRRC elaborates a yellow rust genotyping and race analyses report based on a large number of samples being shipped from around the world. Genotyping was based on single sequence repeat (SSR) analysis and race phenotyping was based on bioassays of differential wheat lines using spore samples of recovered, pure isolates grown under strict experimental conditions (Hovmøller et al., 2019). A clear connection between the unusual epidemics and the incursion of new exotic SR strains into Argentina was evidenced. Genotyping results showed that a single genetic lineage named as *PstS13* was prevalent (80% of the sampled localities) in 2017 (Hovmøller et al., 2018). The testing of additional samples from 2018 confirmed the widespread of *PstS13* as it was completely dominating the composition of genetic lineages determined (100% of the sampled localities in Argentina) (Figure 11). Isolates of *PstS13* were first detected on Triticale giving rise to significant epidemics in Northern Europe in 2015. Later it was detected in Italy, Ukraine, Spain, Poland, Netherlands and three Scandinavian countries. Only a single race has been detected in the *PstS13* lineage in 2017 causing severe epidemics on bread wheat and durum wheat in Italy. Significant yield losses caused by highly aggressive *PstS13* isolates on multiple spring wheat (Carmona et al., 2019) and durum wheat (southern Europe) varieties and multiple triticale varieties (northern Europe and South America) were reported so far (Hovmøller et al., 2019). In 2019, a new *Yr10*-virulent variant in *PstS13* was detected in Europe. In Argentina, although only a single race (virulence phenotype: -,2,-,-,-,6,7,8,9,-,-,-,-,-,-,-,-,AvS,-) has been detected irrespective of sampling origin, the determination of the particular race of *PstS13* is pending.

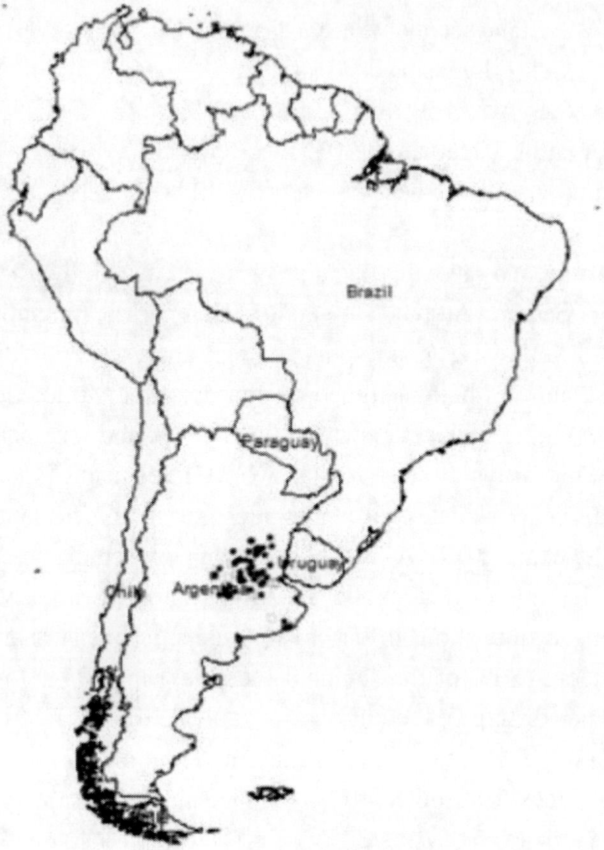

Figure 11a. Location of Argentinean wheat fields in South America sampled for SR epidemic monitoring.

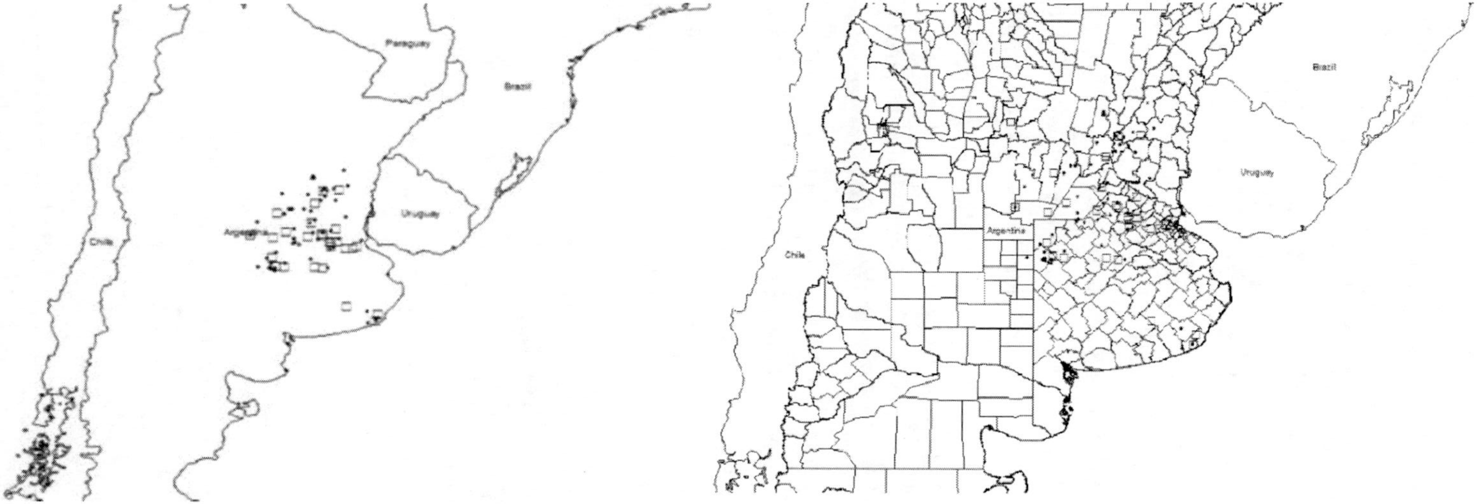

Figure 11b. Location of wheat fields sampled in 2017 (squares) and 2018 (black dots) in Argentina for SR epidemic monitoring.

A different genetic lineage, *PstS14*, first detected in Europe in 2016 and Morocco, Africa in 2017, was also detected in Argentina in 2017 epidemics with a prevalence of 13% (Hovmøller et al., 2018). Further, another genetic lineage harboring the '*Warrior*' race, *PstS7*, was detected in only one sample (2.6% prevalence) in Argentina in 2017. The first confirmation of the detection of this lineage in Argentina in a non-epidemic situation was in 2015. The PstS7 isolates from Argentina (both 2015 and 2017) were unique, diverging by 1-2 alleles from the PstS7 isolates in Europe and West Asia (Hovmøller et al., 2018). These findings are in agreement with the hypothesis proposed by Ali et al. (2014) that Europe could be the source of origin of the SR populations infecting wheat in South America. Isolates of the *PstS13* lineage were detected in 2017 both in Italy and Argentina causing severe epidemics on wheat. The about 12,000 km separation distance between these geographic regions suggests a high global dispersal capacity of *Pst*. However, this hypothesis has yet to be demonstrated at least with dispersion prediction models according to the prevailing global circulation patterns.

An important component in the onset and development of rust epidemics is the role of alternate hosts of *Pst*. To date, however, for the case of SR there is no evidence or relationship that secondary hosts may play a key role in the epidemiology of the disease in Argentina (Carmona et al., 2020), even though SR has been detected in triticale (X Triticosecale), rye (*Secale cereale*) and tricepiro (hexaploid Triticale x octoploid Trigopyre).

Although the information available is not sufficient to fully clarify the epidemiology of the disease in Argentina, we hypothesize that: (i) the recent widespread SR epidemics caused by new aggressive *Pst* strains in Argentina were the result of direct introductions of airborne urediniospores from inoculum source areas in southern Africa, and (ii) the spatio-temporal progress of disease in the wheat growing regions of the country was the result of intermitent spore reintroductions in air parcels or land bridge inoculum accumulation in host areas resulted from short-distance dispersal of spores by surface winds. Research exploring these areas is underway. This analysis paves the way to new studies on control and understanding of the biology of this pathogen.

Preventing SR Epidemics

Wheat SR epidemiology has changed dramatically in Argentina since 2017 in terms of cultivar susceptibility and disease severity. Unlike other regions of the world where SR occurrence has increased during the last 20 years, recent SR epidemics in Argentina were built up over three years and have been the most severe since 1930. It is expected that SR epidemics will continue to occur due to the presence of new SR strains virulent on wheat varieties and because most of the high yield potential wheat cultivars that are planted in the country are highly susceptible to SR. For all this, the risks of SR epidemics and susceptibility response of wheat cultivars to the pathogen strains has become unpredictable for wheat producers and plant breeders.

Integrated management of SR should combine control strategies such as planting SR-resistant wheat varieties, development of local or regional infection risk models to predict SR epidemics, frequent scouting, balanced fertilization, appropriate use of efficacious fungicides (seed and foliar treatment) and development of local or regional decision support tools for timing fungicide applications. It is likely that SR-resistant wheat varieties with appropriate level of durable resistance be developed in the near future. Planting of such varieties should be promoted or encouraged to avoid planting a few varieties with high-yield potential but highly SR-susceptible in the largest proportion of the wheat area. Additionally, it is highly recommended to scout not only SR-susceptible cultivars but also SR-resistant varieties that can be broken down within a few years after their release. Some cultural practices can contribute to the increase of an epidemic if they contribute to create a greater number of infected volunteer plants, vegetating during the period between wheat crops.

The use of fungicides has become one of the most important tools for SR control worldwide, especially when susceptible genotypes are planted. Numerous fungicides formulations are available for SR control in the different wheat growing regions of the world (Carmona et al., 2020). The combination choice of fungicide active ingredients (a.i.), time and rate of application must be defined for each field depending on the level of genetic resistance to SR of the planted wheat variety, the level of disease intensity and the forecast of weather variables conducive to disease development. One of the most important points is the optimal timing for fungicide application according to scientific criteria. Late fungicide applications are ineffective and have a reduced yield economic response. We proposed the development of a local or regional economic damage threshold (EDT). For example, 10–20% of SR foliar incidence from the Z3.0 wheat growth stage is a preliminary guideline in Argentina (Carmona et al., 2019). Following this recommendation, several field trials with fungicides were carried out. During the 2017/2018 growing season, trials were conducted in Landeta, Santa Fe province, with yield responses to fungicide as high as 3091 kg ha^{-1} and 4743 kg ha^{-1} for one and two sprays in susceptible wheat genotypes, respectively. The results indicated that one or two fungicide applications significantly decreased SR intensity and increased the wheat grain yield. In 2019, a field trial was conducted in Bigand, Santa Fe (-35.5963 S, -62.9838 W), in order to determine the effect of different fungicide a.i. efficiency on SR control and its impact on wheat grain yield. Significant differences occurred between treated and untreated plots. One application of Allegro® (kresoxim-methyl 12.5% + epoxiconazole 12.5%) at Z3.1 resulted in 1,323 kg ha^{-1} yield increase. Treatments with two fungicide applications of Allegro® (kresoxim-methyl 12.5% + epoxiconazole 12.5%) + Opera® (pyraclostrobin 13.3% + epoxiconazole 5%) in Z3.1 and Allegro® (kresoxim-methyl 12.5% + epoxiconazole 12.5%) + Orquesta Ultra® (fluxapiroxad 5% + pyraclostrobin 8.1% + epoxiconazole 5%) in Z3.9 controlled > 90% of the SR severity, with a significant yield increase of 2373 and 2217 kg ha^{-1}, respectively, compared to the untreated control. These data confirm the potentially damaging effects of SR in susceptible wheat varieties in Argentina and the high efficacy of different fungicidal active ingredients for its control. Carmona et al. (2020) recently published a comprehensive review of the impact and role of fungicides in the integrated management of SR. This review further summarizes the registered fungicides and timing of foliar spray that are recommended worldwide.

Conclusion

Despite the potential damage that SR can cause in wheat crops in Argentina and elsewhere, and the relatively low cost of fungicides to control the disease effectively, it is likely that Argentina growers will continue to plant high-yield potential, yet highly SR susceptible wheat varieties. Our analysis suggests that to achieve an efficient and complementary management of SR, regional disease early warning system and government programs should be implemented. Efforts must include early monitoring in the growing season, starting in the fields with the highest epidemiological risk, using sentinel plots and weather monitoring. It is emphasized that the quantitative monitoring and image processing of urediniospores efficiently captured from wheat fields could provide critical information for SR prediction (Lei et al., 2018). Further, the need for SR scouting and monitoring for emergence of fungicide resistance are key points to assist growers.

In this review, we have outlined a detailed description of the morphological characteristics that must be recognized for an early diagnosis of SR. Diagnosis should couple visual disease monitoring in wheat crops as well as in volunteer wheat plants where inoculum could cause primary infections early in the growing season. Our extensive work on chemical control of SR and assessments of economic losses indicate that timing detection of SR and weather monitoring are paramount for fungicide application decisions, which are conducive to prevention of disease or reduction of the amount of initial inoculum.

Acknowledgments

The authors thank all the people who have contributed to sampling and submission of rust infected leaves: Carlos Grosso, Diego Alvarez, Gustavo Duarte, Fabricio Mock, Jonathan Damiani, Julián García, Lucrecia Couretot, Marcos Mitelsky, Mariano Vence, Norma Formento, Alejandro Porfiri,

Roxana Maumary, Andrea Rosso, Agustín Bilbao, Agustín Pulido, Ana Rodríguez, Ana Storm, Buck Semillas, Carina Cáceres, Claudio Bosco, Cristina Palacios, Enrique Alberione, Franco Petrelli, Ignacio Erreguerena, Liliana Wehrhahne, Adelina Larsen, Manuela Gordo, Margarita Sillón, Florencia Magliano, Mauro Montarini, Victoria Gonzalez, Daniel Ploper.

REFERENCES

Ali, S., Gladieux, P., Leconte, M., Gautier, A., Justesen, A. F., Hovmøller, M. S., Enjalbert, J., de Vallavieille-Pope, C. (2014). Origin, Migration Routes and Worldwide Population Genetic Structure of the Wheat Yellow Rust Pathogen *Puccinia striiformis* f. sp. *tritici*. *PLoS Pathogens*, 10(1): e1003903. doi: 10.1371/journal.ppat.1003903.

Beddow, J. M., Pardey, P. G., Chai, Y., Hurley, T. M., Kriticos, D. J., Braun, H.-J, Park, R. F., et al. (2015). Research investment implica-tions of shifts in the global geography of wheat stripe rust. *Nature Plants*, 1: 15132. doi: 10.1038/nplants.2015.132.

Bolton, M. D., Kolmer, J. A., Garvin, D. F. (2008). Wheat leaf rust caused by *Puccinia triticina*. *Molecular Plant Pathology*, 9(5): 563-575. doi: 10.1111/j.1364-3703.2008.00487.x.

Brown, J. K. M., Hovmøller, M. (2002). Aerial dispersal of pathogens on the global and continental scales and its impact on plant disease. *Science*, 297: 537–541.

Bushnell, W. R, Roelfs, A. P. (1984), *Origins, Specificity, Structure, and Physiology*. Academic Press. 566 p. doi: 10.1016/B978-0-12-148401-9.X5001-8.

Carmona, M., Sautua, F., Pérez-Hernández, O., Reis, E. M. (2020). Role of fungicide applications on the integrated management of wheat stripe rust. *Frontiers in Plant Science*, 11: 733. doi: 10.3389/fpls.2020.00733.

Carmona, M. A., Sautua, F. J., Pérez-Hernández, O., et al. (2019). Rapid emergency response to yellow rust epidemics caused by newly introduced lineages of *Puccinia striiformis* f. sp. *tritici* in Argentina. *Tropical Plant Pathology*, 44: 385. doi: 10.1007/s40858-019-00295-y.

Carmona, M. A., Reis, E. M., Cortese P. (2000). Wheat rusts. Diagnosis, epidemiology and control strategies. 21 pp. ISBN 987-43-2641-7.

Chen, X. M. (2005). Epidemiology and control of stripe rust [*Puccinia striiformis* f. sp. *tritici*] on wheat. *Canadian Journal of Plant Pathology*, 27: 314–37. doi: 10.1080/07060660509507230.

Chen, W., Wellings, C., Chen, X., Kang, Z., Liu, T. (2014). Wheat stripe (yellow) rust caused by *Puccinia striiformis* f. sp. *tritici*. *Molecular Plant Pathology*, 15(5): 433-446. doi: 10.1111/mpp.12116.

Chen, X. M., Kang, Z. (2017a). *Introduction: History of Research, Symptoms, Taxonomy of the Pathogen, Host Range, Distribution, and Impact of Stripe Rust*. In: Chen, X. M. & Z. Zang (Eds.). Stripe Rust. Springer Netherlands. pp. 1-33. doi: 10.1007/978-94-024-1111-9.

Chen, X. M. (2020). Pathogens which threaten food security: *Puccinia striiformis*, the wheat stripe rust pathogen. *Food Security*, 12: 239–251. doi: 10.1007/s12571-020-01016-z.

Eriksson, J., Henning, E. (1896). *The cereal rusts.* Nortstedt & Söner, Stockholm.

Farber, D. H., Medlock, J., Mundt, C. C. (2017). Local dispersal of *Puccinia striiformis* f. sp. *tritici* from isolated source lesions. *Plant pathology* 66(1): 28–37. doi: 10.1111/ppa.12554.

Fernandez Valiela, M. V. 1979. *Introduction to Phytopathology.* Vol. IV: Hongos y Mycoplasmas. Colección Científica INTA. 3a Edición. Buenos Aires. República Argentina. 613 pp.

Geagea, L. W., Huber, L., Sache, I. (1997). Removal of urediniospores of brown (*Puccinia recondita* f. sp. *tritici*) and yellow (*Puccinia striiformis*) rusts of wheat from infected leaves submitted to a mechanical stress. *European Journal of Plant Pathology*, 103: 785–793. doi: 10.1023/A:1008629328161.

Geagea, L., Huber, L., Sache, I. (1999). Dry-dispersal and rain-splash of brown (*Puccinia recondita* f. sp. *tritici*) and yellow (*P. striiformis*) rust spores from infected wheat leaves exposed to simulated raindrops. *Plant Pathology*, 48: 472-482. doi: 10.1046/j.1365-3059.1999.00372.x.

Germán, S., Barcellos, A., Chaves, M., Kohli, M., Campos, P., de Viedma, L. (2007). The situation of common wheat rusts in the Southern Cone of America and perspectives for control. *Australian Journal of Agricultural Research*, 58: 620-630. doi: 10.1071/AR06149.

Hovmøller, M. S., Justesen, A. F., and Brown, J. K. M. (2002). Clonality and long-distance migration of *Puccinia striiformis* f. sp. *tritici* in north-west Europe. *Plant Pathology*, 51: 24–32. doi: 10.1046/j.1365-3059.2002.00652.x.

Hovmøller, M. S., Walter, S., Justesen, A. F. 2010. Escalating Threat of Wheat Rusts. *Science*, 329: 369. doi: 10.1126/science.1194925.

Hovmøller, M. S., Rodriguez-Algaba, J., Thach, T., Justesen, A. F., Hansen, J. G. 2018. *Report for Puccinia striiformis race analyses and molecular genotyping 2017,* Global Rust Reference Center (GRRC), Aarhus University, available at: http://wheatrust.org/fileadmin/www.grcc.au.dk/International_Services/Pathotype_YR_results/Summary_of_Puccinia_striiformis_race_analysis_2017.pdf (accesed 18 July 2020).

Hovmøller, M. S., Rodriguez-Algaba, J., Thach, T., Justesen, A. F., Hansen, J. G. 2019. *GRRC Annual report 2019: Stem- and yellow rust genotyping and race analyses.* Available at: https://agro.au.dk/fileadmin/www.grcc.au.dk/International_Services/Pathotype_YR_results/GRRC_annual_report_2019.pdf (accesed 14 July 2020).

Huang, S., Zuo, S., Zheng, D. et al. 2019. Three formae speciales of *Puccinia striiformis* were identified as heteroecious rusts based on completion of sexual cycle on *Berberis* spp. under artificial inoculation. *Phytopathology Research*, 1: 14. doi: 10.1186/s42483-019-0021-y.

Humphrey, H. B., Cromwell, R. O. 1930. Stripe rust (*Puccinia glumarum*) on wheat in Argentina. *Phytopathology*, 20: 981-986.

Leonard, K. J., Szabo, L. J. (2005). Stem rust of small grains and grasses caused by *Puccinia graminis*. *Molecular Plant Pathology*, 6(2): 99-111. doi: 10.1111/j.1364-3703.2005.00273.x.

Lei, Y., Yao, Z., He, D. (2018). Automatic detection and counting of urediniospores of *Puccinia striiformis* f. sp. *tritici* using spore traps and image processing. *Scientific Reports*, 8: 13647. doi: 10.1038/s41598-018-31899-0.

Lindquist, J. C., 1982. *Rusts of the Argentine Republic and bordering areas.* Colección científica del INTA. 574 p.

Mehmood, S., Sajid, M., Huang, L., Kang, Z. (2020a). Alternate hosts and their impact on genetic diversity of *Puccinia striiformis* f. sp. *tritici* and disease epidemics. *Journal of Plant Interactions*, 15: 153-165, doi: 10.1080/17429145.2020.1771445.

Mehmood, S., Sajid, M., Zhao, J., Huang, L., Kang, Z. (2020b). Alternate hosts of *Puccinia striiformis* f. sp. *tritici* and their role. *Pathogens*, 9(6): 434. doi: 10.3390/pathogens9060434.

MINAGRI. Ministry of Agriculture, Livestock and Fisheries. *Agricultural statistics.* 2018. http://datosestimaciones.magyp.gob.ar/

Rapilly, F. (1979). Yellow Rust Epidemiology. *Annual Review of Phytopathology*, 17(1): 59–73. doi: 10.1146/annurev.py.17.090179.000423.

Roelfs, A. P. (1985). Wheat and rye stem rust. pp. 3–37. In: Roelfs, A. P., Bushnell, W. R. (eds.), *The Cereal Rusts Vol. II: Diseases, Distribution, Epidemiology, and Control.* Orlando, FL: Academic.

Roelfs, A. P., Singh, R. P., Saari, E. E. 1992. *Rust Diseases of Wheat: Concepts and methods of disease management.* Mexico, D.F.: CIMMYT. 81 pages.

Rudorf, W., Job, M. 1934. Studies regarding the specialization of *Puccinia graminis tritici. Puccinia trilicina* and *Puccinia glumarum tritici*, as well as on resistance and its inheritance in different crosses. *Plant breeding* 19: 333-365.

Schwessinger, B. (2016). Fundamental wheat stripe rust research in the 21st century. *New Phytologist*, 213: 1625–1631. doi: 10.1111/nph.14159.

Stubbs, R. W. 1985. Stripe rust. In: Roelfs, A. P. y W. R. Bushnell (Eds.). *The Cereal Rusts, Diseases, Distribution, Epidemiology and Control.* London, UK: Academic Press. pp. 61–101.

Wang, M. N, Chen, X. M. (2013). First report of Oregon Grape (*Mahonia aquifolium*) as an alternate host for the wheat stripe rust pathogen (*Puccinia striiformis* f. sp. *tritici*) under artificial inoculation. *Plant Disease*, 97(6): 839. doi: 10.1094/PDIS-09-12-0864-PDN.

Wellings, C. R. (2007). *Puccinia striiformis* in Australia: A review of the incursion, evolution and adaptation of stripe rust in the period 1979-2006. *Australian Journal of Agricultural Research*, 58: 567-575.

Zhao, J., Wang, M., Chen, X., Kang, Z. (2016). Role of alternate hosts in epidemiology and pathogen variation of cereal rusts. *Annual Review of Phytopathology*, 54: 207-228. doi: 10.1146/annurev-phyto-080615-095851.

INDEX

A

B

C

D

E

F

G

H

I

L

M

N

O

P

R

S

T

V

W

Y

A